Cardiac Diseases and Interventions in 21st Century

Edited by Ozgur Karcioglu

Published in London, United Kingdom

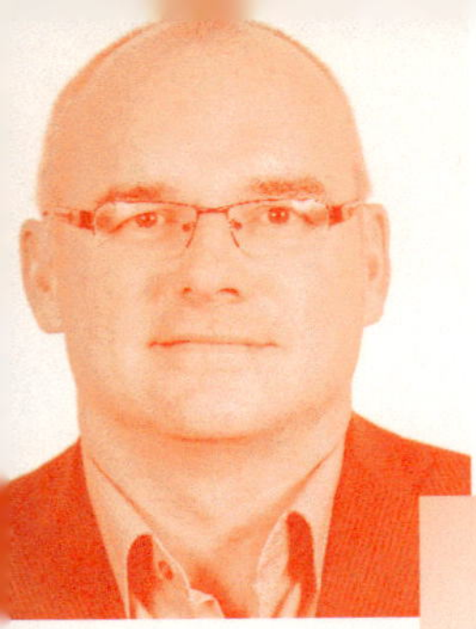
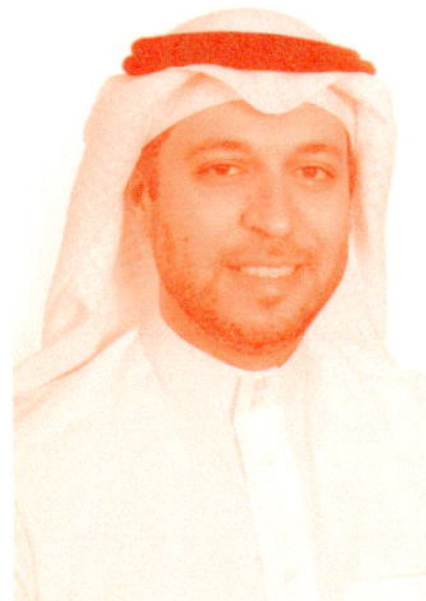
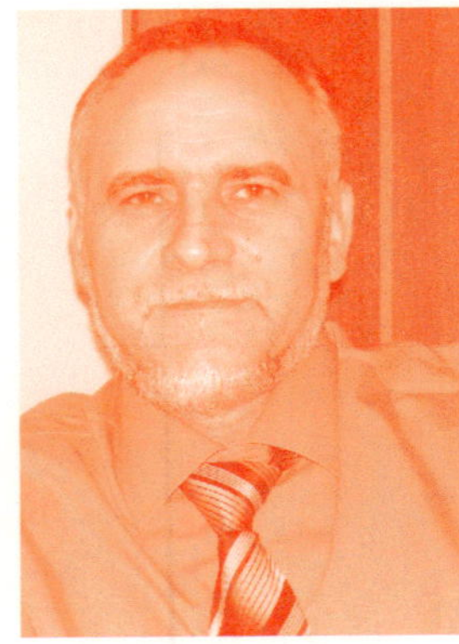
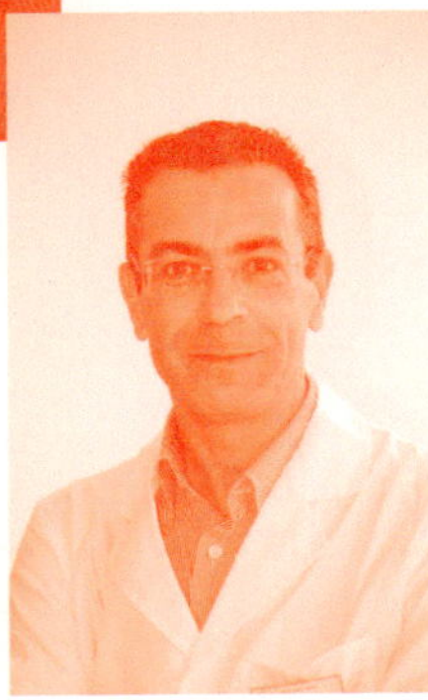
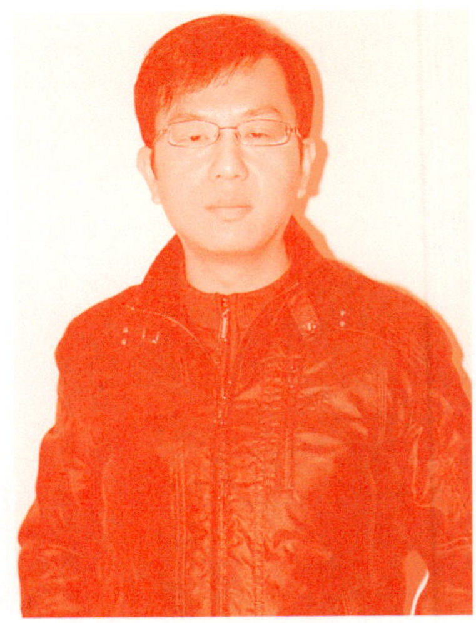
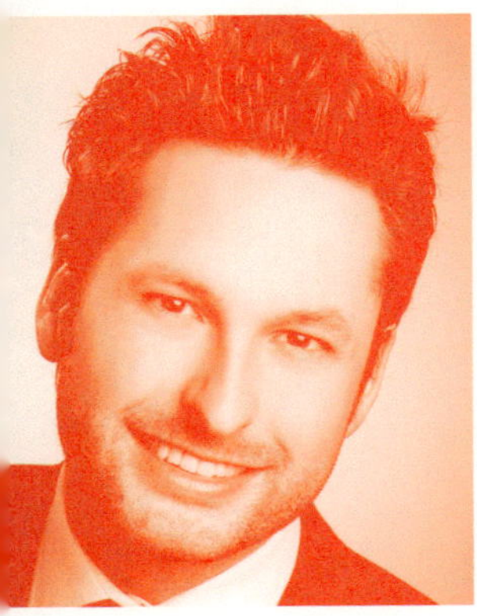
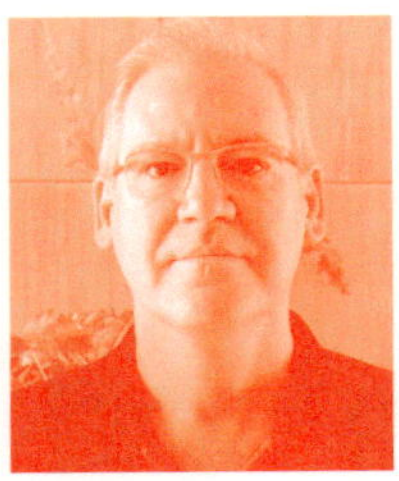

IntechOpen

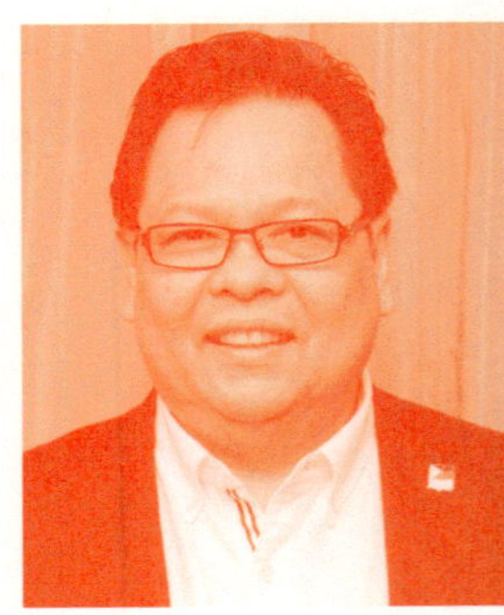
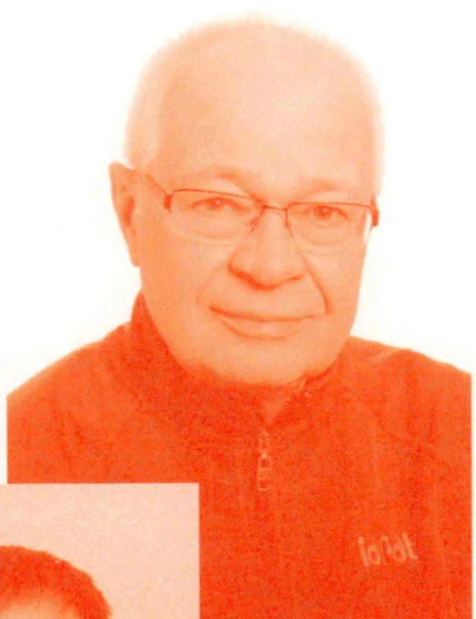
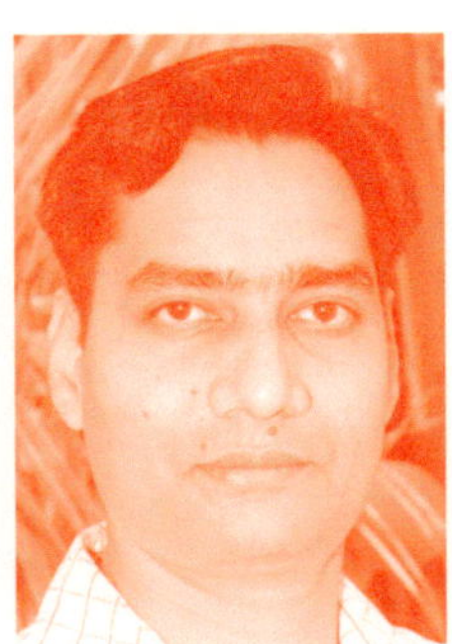
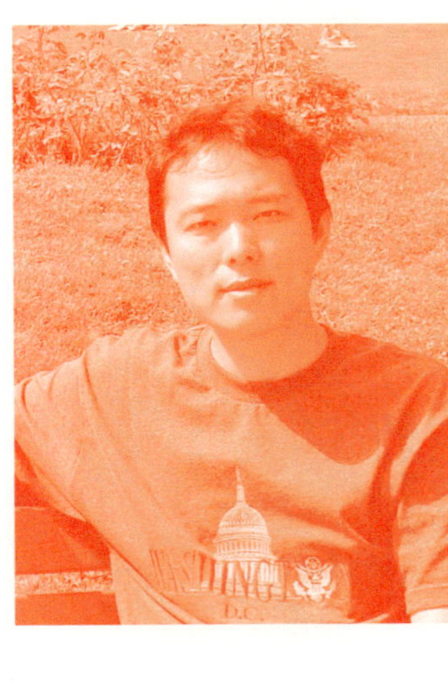
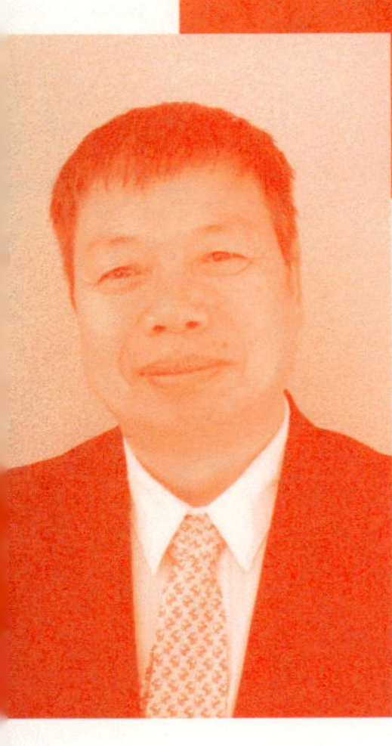
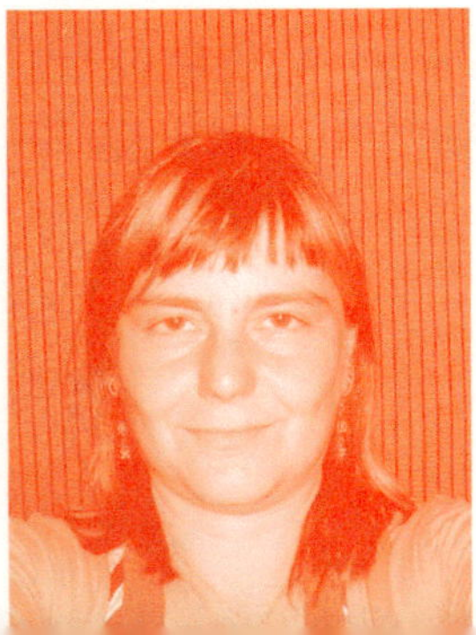

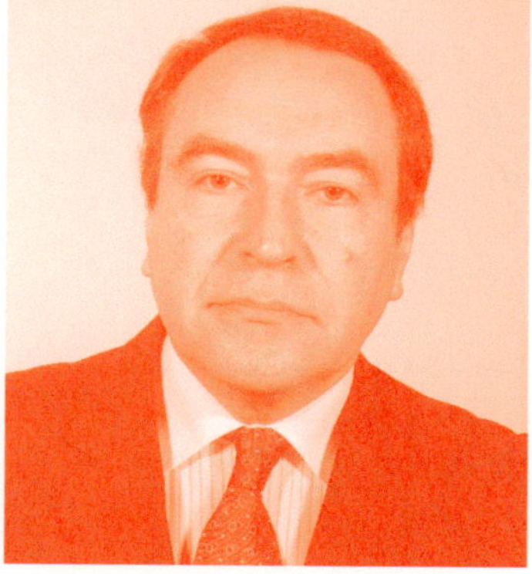

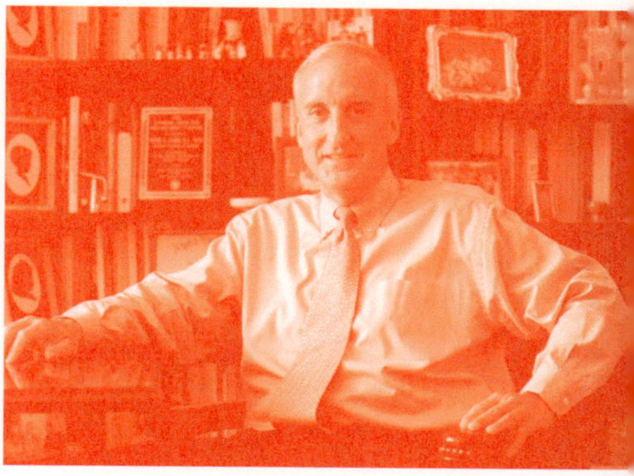

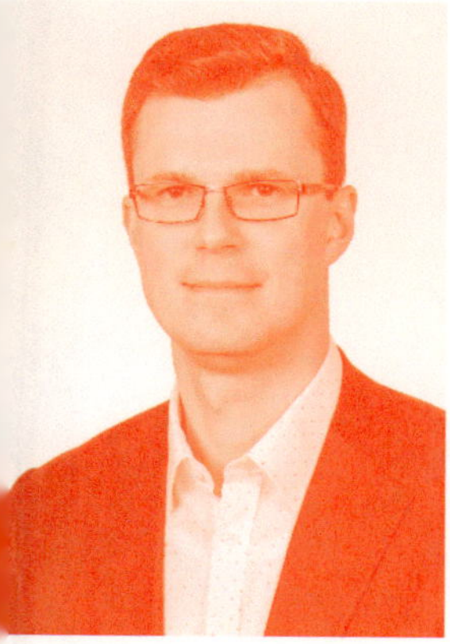

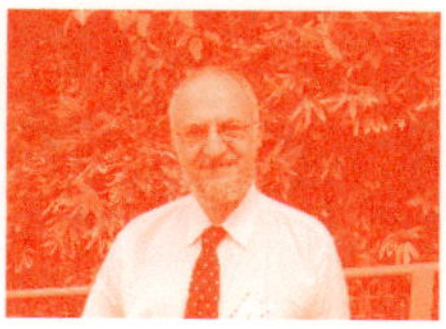

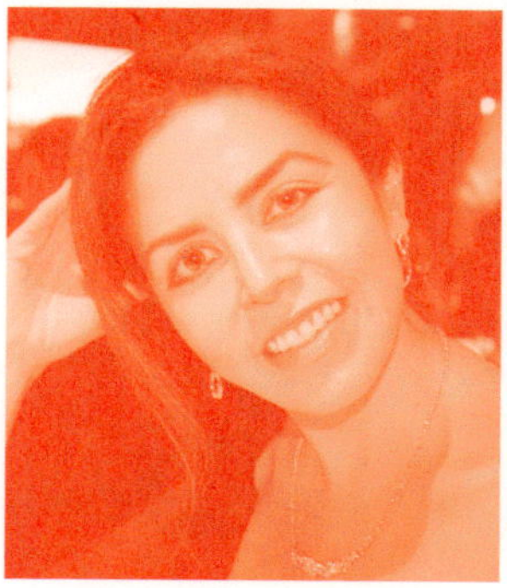

Supporting open minds since 2005

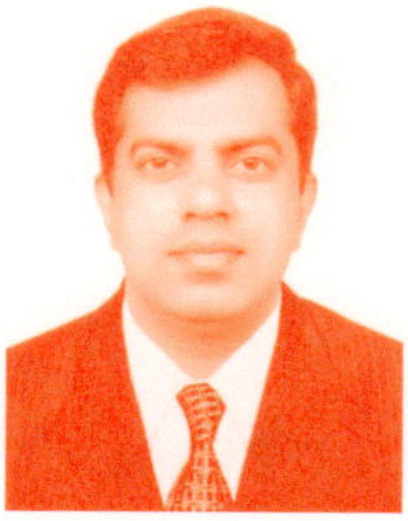

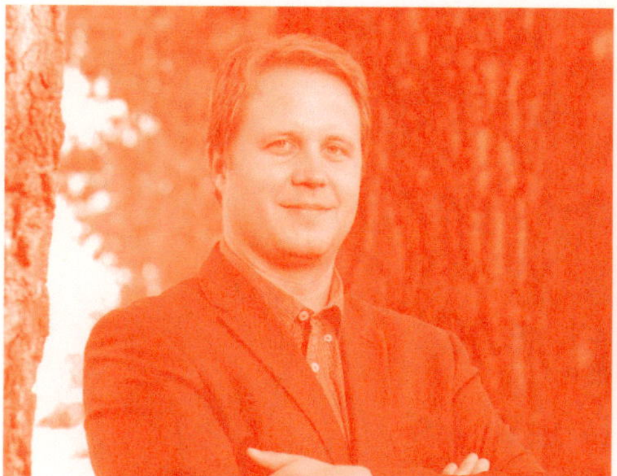

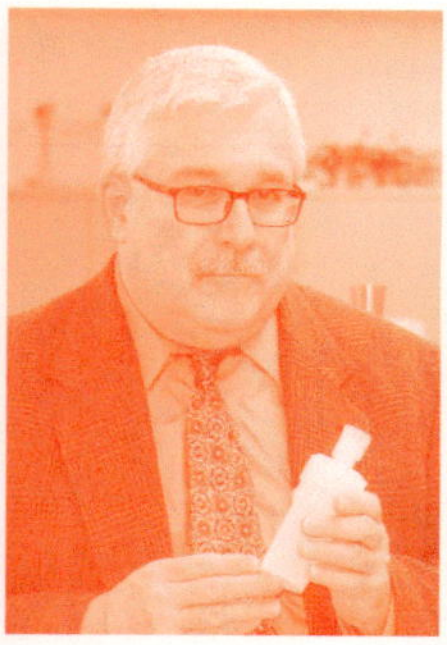

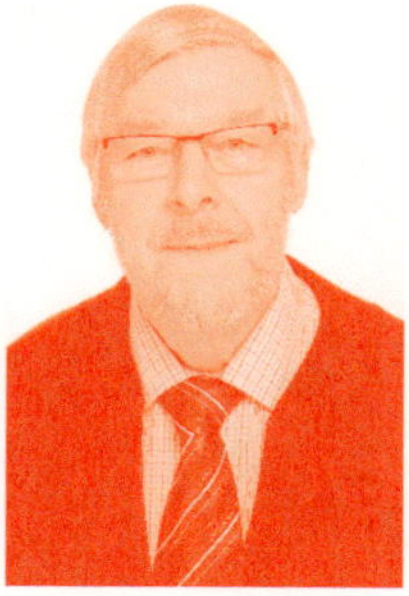

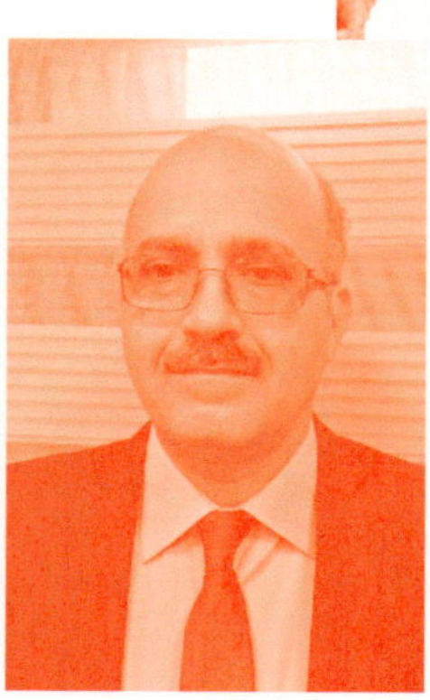

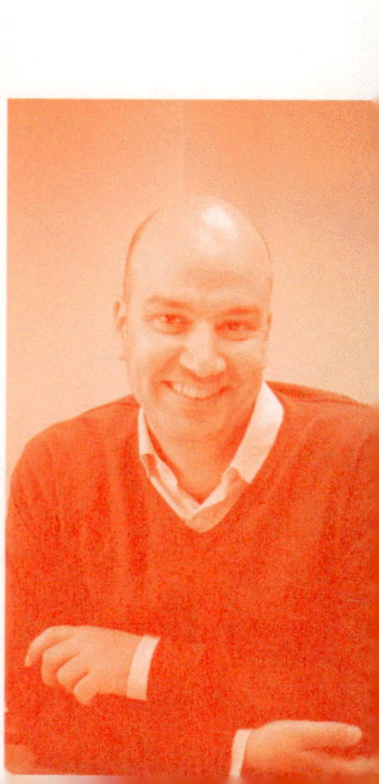

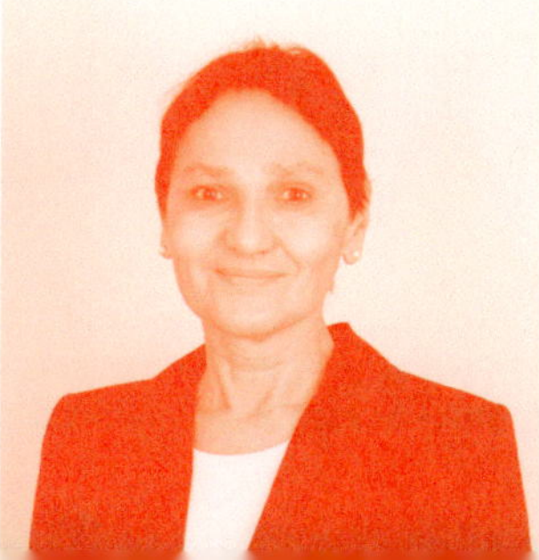

Cardiac Diseases and Interventions in 21st Century
http://dx.doi.org/10.5772/intechopen.78250
Edited by Ozgur Karcioglu

Contributors
Ruslan Linchak, Sergey Boytsov, Andrey Ardashev, Artem Kuzovlev, Gulnora Nagaeva, David Wieczorek, Mikel Leturiondo, Sofia Ruiz De Gauna, Jose Julio Gutierrez, Digna M González-Otero, Jesus Ruiz, Luis Alberto Leturiondo, Purificacion Saiz, Jean-Marc Mercantini, Dan Blendea, Sabina Istratoaie, Mirela-Anca Stoia, Sorin Pop, Florin Anton, Sorin Crisan, Ozgur KARCIOGLU

First published in London, United Kingdom, 2019 by IntechOpen
IntechOpen is the global imprint of INTECHOPEN LIMITED, registered in England and Wales, registration number: 11086078, The Shard, 25th floor, 32 London Bridge Street
London, SE19SG – United Kingdom
Printed in Croatia

British Library Cataloguing-in-Publication Data
A catalogue record for this book is available from the British Library

Additional hard and PDF copies can be obtained from orders@intechopen.com

Cardiac Diseases and Interventions in 21st Century
Edited by Ozgur Karcioglu
p. cm.
Print ISBN 978-1-83881-990-3
Online ISBN 978-1-83881-991-0
eBook (PDF) ISBN 978-1-83881-992-7

For EU product safety concerns:
IN TECH d.o.o., Prolaz Marije Krucifikse Kozulić 3, 51000 Rijeka, Croatia, info@intechopen.com or visit our website at intechopen.com.

Meet the editor

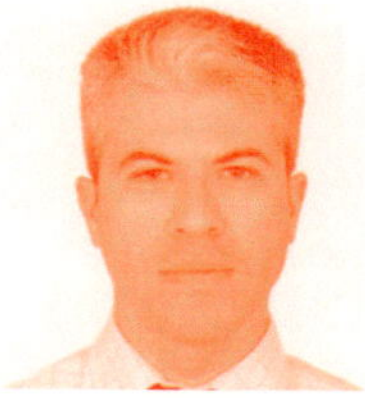

Dr. Ozgur Karcioglu graduated from his residency at Dokuz Eylul University Medical School, Department of Emergency Medicine, Turkey, in 1998. He attended the "International Emergency Medicine" Fellowship in Penn State University (2005) and now he is the Chair of the Department of Emergency Medicine, Istanbul Education and Research Hospital.

He served as a founder and board member of The Emergency Medical Association of Turkey since 1995. He has had more than 130 articles published in scientific journals, has contributed to five books as editor, and authored 35 chapters. Recently, he has published *Trauma Surgery* and *Poisoning in the Modern World* with the collaboration of IntechOpen. He is also an instructor of the Advanced Cardiac Life Support Course.

Contents

Preface **XI**

Section 1
Introduction **1**

Chapter 1 **3**
Introductory Chapter: Cardiac Disease - Plague in the Modern World
by Ozgur Karcioglu

Section 2
Monitoring, Investigations and Simulations in Training **7**

Chapter 2 **9**
The Role of Tropomyosin in Cardiac Function and Disease
by David F. Wieczorek

Chapter 3 **23**
Waveform Capnography for Monitoring Ventilation during Cardiopulmonary Resuscitation: The Problem of Chest Compression Artifact
by Mikel Leturiondo, Sofía Ruiz de Gauna, José Julio Gutiérrez, Digna M. González-Otero, Jesus M. Ruiz, Luis A. Leturiondo and Purificación Saiz

Chapter 4 **43**
Characteristics of Acute Myocardial Damage in Uzbekistan: Data Register "RACSMI-Uz"
by Nagaeva Gulnora

Chapter 5 **69**
Ontology-Based Modeling for Newborn Behavior Simulation during Cardiopulmonary Resuscitation
by Jean-Marc Mercantini

Section 3
Treatment and Interventions **91**

Chapter 6 **93**
The Importance of Lead Positioning to Improve Clinical Outcomes in Cardiac Resynchronization Therapy
by Mirela-Anca Stoia, Sabina Istratoaie, Sorin Pop, Florin Anton, Sorin Crisan and Dan Blendea

Chapter 7 109
Public-Access Defibrillation in Sudden Cardiac Arrest
by Ruslan Linchak, Sergey Boytsov, Andrey Ardashev and Artem Kuzovlev

Preface

The optimal management of patients with cardiac disease warrants a multifaceted approach undertaken in harmony. Recent decades have witnessed major advances in methods for monitoring and interventions aimed at improving outcomes in this outstanding cause of death worldwide. Other than technological improvements, the medical community is aware that this task can only be achieved via a mutual collaboration of actors in prehospital phase, hospital emergency departments, intensive care units, social studies, public health professionals, and bystanders. In brief, only those targeted people that could be reached via awareness programs can make a difference in this context.

This book is intended to encompass the advancements in diagnoses and treatment modalities for cardiac diseases in general, and emergency cardiac conditions in particular.

Ozgur Karcioglu, MD, FEMAT
Professor,
Department of Emergency Medicine,
University of Health Sciences,
Istanbul Education and Research Hospital,
Fatih, Istanbul, Turkey

Section 1

Introduction

Chapter 1

Introductory Chapter: Cardiac Disease - Plague in the Modern World

Ozgur Karcioglu

1. Introduction

Medicine has been recognized as an art of understanding and healing human illnesses and injuries for thousands of years. Warfare, economic turmoils, and all kinds of socioeconomic factors affect medical knowledge and practice in cardiac diseases, mostly prominent in the last centuries.

After 1960s, breakthrough changes and innovations in cardiac biomarkers, electrocardiographic monitoring, defibrillation, therapeutic temperature management (TTM), capnography, and some other instruments have been launched, and these have been thought to mitigate the burden of cardiac diseases. Nowadays, it is obvious that electrocardiography, defibrillation, and cardiopulmonary resuscitation (CPR) are far from its current format in the 1950's and 1960's world.

Out-of-hospital cardiac arrest (OHCA) remains a major death scenario in the middle-aged population all over the world. Despite all new major advances, survival for OHCA is, on average, approximately 10%, but substantial variability is visible among emergency medical services systems even in the most developed countries. Four kinds of fatal arrhythmias (ventricular fibrillation-VF, pulseless ventricular tachycardia, asystole, and pulseless electrical activity) result in a loss of cardiac function and sudden cardiac death.

VF is one of the most deadly cardiac arrhythmias and certainly the most common one. It can be described as erratic, disorganized firing of impulses from the ventricles, producing no palpable pulses in the periphery. Literature data have shown that the earlier defibrillation and bystander CPR have been commenced, the lower is the patient mortality. Since considerable differences can affect people's lives in this context, the role of medical command bears utmost importance to direct these patients to facilities with discrete capabilities [1].

Another aspect of the emergency life-saving interventions in these patients comprises **urgent coronary revascularization.** Since most patients presenting with OHCA and refractory VF suffer from an acute thrombotic coronary artery lesion, urgent coronary angiography with revascularization is critical.

1.1 Alternative approaches to VF

Although the majority of patients with refractory VF do not respond to conventional therapy, recent trials of novel strategies demonstrate encouraging results [2]. For example, some recent reports pointed out that **double sequential defibrillation** can be a viable alternative to the classical approaches for the management of shock-refractory VF [3]. Certainly, further study is warranted before widespread practice of this technique.

Recent advances in extracorporeal life support and point-of-care ultrasound imaging, both in-hospital and out-of-hospital, may offer a therapeutic solution in some systems for patients with refractory cardiac arrest rhythms. Similarly, modern improvizations have brought drones into use to fetch automated external defibrillators to the scene of an OHCA, advances in digital and mobile techniques to improve bystander response, and wearable life detection technologies may increase survival [4].

Creating a system of care for OHCA is challenging the medical community. It must be a multifaceted approach that encompasses a variety of teams from call takers, to bystanders, to emergency medical service (EMS) personnel, and to hospital personnel [5]. Implementation of these concepts in one's system of care for OHCA will result in a greater number of survivors returning to reproductive life.

Most of the up-to-date treatment recommendations for increasing survival from cardiac arrest revolve around improving the quality of CPR. A focus on delivering therapeutic techniques proved useful and administration of these treatments reliably, using measurement, monitoring, and implementation of quality-improvement strategies, will provide a basis, and in this way, future developments in resuscitation care can be contemplated [6].

As a result of these fundamental developments, post-cardiac arrest syndrome has been intrigued in more detail. Namely, therapeutic temperature management is becoming the standard of care in most institutions in order to give the highest chance of recovery without major sequelae after return of spontaneous circulation [7].

2. New horizons

2.1 Therapeutic temperature management

TTM has been trying to improve survival of cardiac arrest patients in the modern medicine, with contradicting results for decades. Following the successful resuscitation, TTM is postulated to mitigate neurologic damage by reducing cerebral oxygen consumption and biochemical damage. Through a variety of mechanisms, TH affects several pathways at the same time to alleviate death rate of the brain cells in OHCA [8, 9]. In brief, worldwide recognized committees for resuscitation recommend continuation of TTM for at least 24 h after achievement of targeted temperature (33–36°C).

2.2 Mechanized devices

The quality of CPR is probably one of the hottest topics for the medical community. This context, comprising chest compression rate, depth, and fraction of hands-on time, is integral to cardiac arrest survival. Some recent data postulated that introducing mechanized devices to target these measures of quality in the challenging prehospital environment may offer better outcomes [10]. Manual chest compressions remain the standard of care; however, in circumstances where high-quality manual chest compressions are difficult or unsafe, paramedics should consider using a mechanical device [11]. By combining high-quality manual chest compressions and judicious application of mechanical chest compressions, EMS agencies can optimize personnel safety and outcomes in OHCA.

Although animal models deliver favorable results on markers of perfusion and manikin studies demonstrate improved consistency of high-quality CPR performance with device use, real-world application of these devices via prospective randomized human researches failed to demonstrate beneficial effects in outcomes and, therefore, cannot be supported by current evidence [10].

2.3. Extracorporeal membrane oxygenation (ECMO)

Recent data derived from well-designed controlled studies suggest that early initiation of ECMO in these patients is critical. In the last decade, outstanding international committees on resuscitation recommended consideration of ECMO in patients presenting with cardiac arrest from presumed reversible etiology, including myocardial infarction, pulmonary embolism, and refractory VF [12].

3. Conclusion

While cardiac disease, specifically acute cardiac catastrophes like VF remains a major death cause for the reproductive age of human being, a multifaceted approach would fit best to improve survival in those with cardiac arrest and other emergencies. This book was intended to focus on the new opportunities for diagnosing cardiac events and for optimal resuscitation of these, in order to save more lives as possible.

Author details

Ozgur Karcioglu
Department of Emergency Medicine, University of Health Sciences, Istanbul Education and Research Hospital, Fatih, Istanbul, Turkey

*Address all correspondence to: okarcioglu@gmail.com

References

[1] Stoecklein HH, Youngquist ST. The role of medical direction in systems of out-of-hospital cardiac arrest. Cardiology Clinics. 2018;**36**(3):409-417

[2] Bell SM, Lam DH, Kearney K, Hira RS. Management of refractory ventricular fibrillation (Prehospital and Emergency Department). Cardiology Clinics. 2018;**36**(3):395-408

[3] Simon EM, Tanaka K. Double sequential defibrillation. Cardiology Clinics. 2018;**36**(3):387-393

[4] Latimer AJ, McCoy AM, Sayre MR. Emerging and future technologies in out-of-hospital cardiac arrest care. Cardiology Clinics. 2018;**36**(3):429-441

[5] McCoy AM. Ten steps to improve cardiac arrest survival in your community. Cardiology Clinics. 2018;**36**(3):335-342

[6] Reed-Schrader E, Rivers WT, White LJ, Clemency BM. Cardiopulmonary resuscitation quality issues. Cardiology Clinics. 2018;**36**(3):351-356

[7] Walker AC, Johnson NJ. Critical care of the post-cardiac arrest patient. Cardiology Clinics. 2018;**36**(3):419-428

[8] Hypothermia After Cardiac Arrest Study Group. Mild therapeutic hypothermia to improve the neurologic outcome after cardiac arrest. The New England Journal of Medicine. 2002;**346**(8):549-556

[9] Karcioglu O. Overview of the use of therapeutic hypothermia in patients resuscitated from cardiac arrest. Journal of Anesthesia and Intensive Care Medicine. 2018;**5**(5):555672

[10] Nordeen CA. Manual versus mechanical cardiopulmonary resuscitation: A case against the machine. Cardiology Clinics. 2018;**36**(3):375-386

[11] Dyson K, Stub D, Bernard S, Smith K. Controversial issues: Pro mechanical cardiopulmonary resuscitation. Cardiology Clinics. 2018;**36**(3):367-374

[12] Link MS, Berkow LC, Kudenchuk PJ, et al. Part 7: Adult advanced cardiovascular life support: 2015 American Heart Association Guidelines update for cardiopulmonary resuscitation and emergency cardiovascular care. Circulation. 2015;**132**(18 Suppl. 2):S444-S464

Section 2

Monitoring, Investigations and Simulations in Training

Chapter 2

The Role of Tropomyosin in Cardiac Function and Disease

David F. Wieczorek

Abstract

Phosphorylation of cardiac sarcomeric proteins plays a major role in the regulation of physiological performance of the heart. Tropomyosin, an essential thin filament protein, regulates muscle contraction and relaxation through its interactions with actin, myosin, and the troponin complex. Studies demonstrate that changes in tropomyosin phosphorylation occur both postpartum and in response to cardiac hypertrophy and heart failure. To address the significance of tropomyosin phosphorylation on cardiac function, we conducted experiments to ascertain the effects of constitutive pseudophosphorylation, dephosphorylation, and dephosphorylation in hypertrophic cardiomyopathic hearts. Recent work demonstrates that pseudophosphorylation of tropomyosin results in dilated cardiomyopathy. Tropomyosin dephosphorylation results in a compensated or physiological cardiac hypertrophic phenotype. In addition, we demonstrated that tropomyosin dephosphorylation phenotypically rescues hearts undergoing cardiac hypertrophy. In summary, these studies collectively demonstrate a significant biological and physiological role for tropomyosin phosphorylation under both normal and cardiomyopathic conditions.

Keywords: tropomyosin, contractile protein phosphorylation, physiological hypertrophy, heart disease

1. Introduction

The cardiovascular system plays an essential role in the viability of all vertebrate organisms by supplying oxygen and nutrients to the cells and tissues of the body and removing carbon dioxide. Because the demands of the body change rapidly, the heart must be able to respond and adapt to ever-changing environments that it confronts on a daily basis, such as developmental changes, physiological pressures, and chemical stimuli. One mechanism that is utilized by the heart is employing multiple contractile protein isoforms that can alter cardiac function under different conditions. Myosin heavy and light chains, skeletal and cardiac actin, the troponin complex, and α- and β-tropomyosin are contractile proteins that have multiple isoforms that are normally differentially expressed in the developing or adult heart. However, these changes in isoform expression during development usually occur over a time period of days to weeks. To respond to more rapidly changing conditions, such as acute stress, a faster and reversible mechanism is warranted to alter protein function, such as protein phosphorylation. The focus of this article is to address the role tropomyosin phosphorylation plays in cardiac function and to illustrate what we have learned about sarcomeric performance from these studies.

2. Tropomyosin expression and phosphorylation in the heart

Tropomyosin (Tpm) is encoded by four distinct genes, with each gene generating multiple isoforms through alternative splicing [1, 2]. These isoforms exhibit developmental and tissue-/cell-specific regulation by the production of striated and smooth muscle, brain, and cytoskeletal/nonmuscle mRNAs and proteins. There are three major striated muscle Tpm isoforms, referred to here as α-Tpm, β-Tpm, and γ-Tpm. The associated striated muscle Tpm proteins exhibit an alpha-helical coiled-coil dimer structure that exists as either homo- or heterodimers. Cummins and Perry [3] and Izumo et al. [4] found that the myocardium of adult small mammals expresses striated muscle α-Tpm, while fetal heart tissue expresses both α- and β-Tpm isoforms. In a more detailed analysis, we determined that the striated muscle-specific β-Tpm isoform is constitutively expressed in murine embryoid bodies during embryogenesis *in utero* [5]. However, the striated muscle α-Tpm isoform is not present until the day 5 embryoid body and the day 7.5 post coitus embryo. Further analyses show that both the striated muscle α- and β-Tpm isoforms are expressed during cardiogenesis (day 11–19 embryonic hearts), with the α-Tpm transcripts becoming the predominant Tpm isoform in the adult mouse heart [5]. The ratio of striated muscle α- to β-Tpm mRNAs changes from 5:1 to 60:1 as the mouse myocardium transitions from an embryonic to an adult state. γ-Tpm is expressed in slow-twitch skeletal musculature, but is not found in the heart. In addition, a cardiac specific α-Tpm isoform, called Tpm1κ, is expressed in humans and other select organisms [6, 7].

Tpm, an α-helical coiled-coil protein dimer, plays an essential role in the regulation of contraction and relaxation in the thin filament of the sarcomere. Tpm regulates contractile activity through its interactions with actin and the troponin complex in the sarcomere. During muscle relaxation when cytoplasmic levels of calcium are low, Tpm blocks the myosin-binding site on the filamentous striated muscle actin. Upon stimulation, cytosolic calcium concentrations increase and bind to troponin C which, through its association with troponin T and I, mediates a conformational change in the Tpm position on actin. This repositioning of Tpm on actin exposes the myosin-binding site. Myosin binds to actin and triggers muscle contractile activity until the stimulation ceases, and calcium is resequestered into the sarcoplasmic reticulum.

Phosphorylation is a major regulator of cardiac function by affecting numerous membrane, cytoplasmic, and sarcomeric proteins. Alterations in the phosphorylation of contractile proteins, such as troponin I, myosin-binding protein C, and the regulatory light chains can affect myofilament calcium sensitivity and to physiologically regulate cardiac function [8–12]. Previous investigations established that Tpm is phosphorylated at serine 283, the penultimate amino acid of the protein (**Figures 1** and **2**) [13–17].

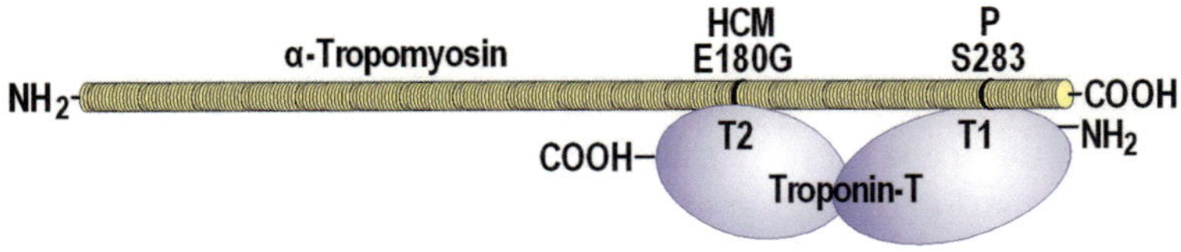

Figure 1.
Diagram of the HCM Tpm180 mutation and the Tpm phosphorylation site. Diagramed in the figure is α-Tpm and the regions where TnT binds Tpm. The number above the Tpm molecule represents the amino acid residues where the hypertrophic cardiomyopathy (HCM) mutation is found and the position of the serine amino acid that is phosphorylated in Tpm.

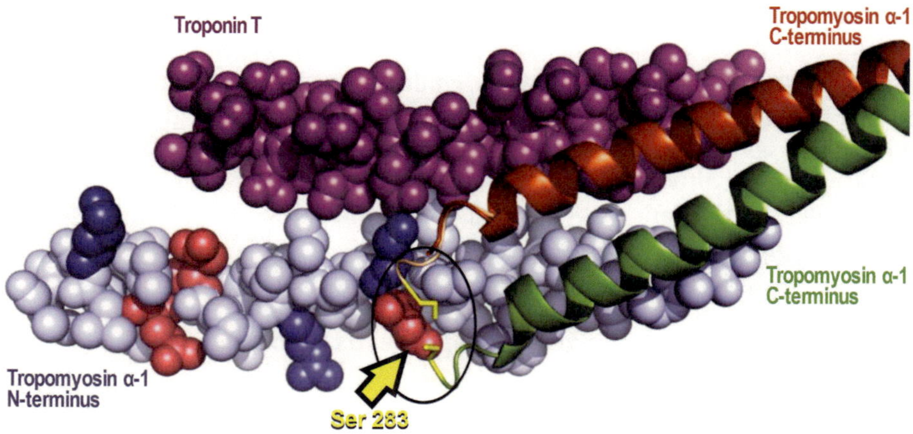

Figure 2.
Model of the Ser283 residues at the C-terminus of tropomyosin. C-terminal Tpm α-1 peptides are shown in dark red and green, troponin T is purple, and the N-terminal Tpm α-1 peptide is shown in gray (adapted from PDB code 2Z5H [18]). Ser283 residues are shown as yellow sticks, highlighted by the black oval. Residues in the Tpm α-1 N-terminal peptide that are positively (blue) or negatively (red) charged are highlighted. Of the two C-terminal Tpm α-1 peptides in the 2Z5H structure, one shows electron density straight through Ser283 (green helix), while the other only shows density through Met281 (dark red helix). Thus, the six C-terminal residues from the complete helix were superimposed on the incomplete helix to illustrate the putative position of Ser283 on this chain (tan extension). Note that in this model, only 1 TnT molecule is present.

This region of Tpm, specifically the carboxyl terminus, plays a critical role in its interaction with actin and troponin T (TnT), and its ability to facilitate polymerization with other Tpm molecules in a head-to-tail fashion [19–21]. Tpm phosphorylation may play a role in increasing the actin-activated myosin S1 ATPase activity, and increase the bond duration between actin-myosin interactions [22, 23]. Thus, phosphorylated Tpm may have an allosteric effect on actin to modify the actin-myosin interaction between the blocked, closed, and open states [24, 25]. Furthermore, the Tpm carboxyl region interacts with TnT, and work by our laboratory demonstrates this region dramatically affects cardiac function by regulating rates of contraction and relaxation, in addition to influencing myofilament calcium sensitivity [26]. The specific role that Tpm phosphorylation plays in influencing the physiological role of the carboxyl terminus and its interactions with the other contractile proteins in determining cardiac function was the subject of our investigations [14, 27, 28], and is being addressed in our current work [29].

The serine residue at amino acid 283 is the phosphorylation site found in the three striated muscle Tpm isoforms. With respect to Tpm phosphorylation, this posttranslational process is developmentally regulated, with 60–70% phosphorylated α-Tpm being present in the murine heart during fetal and newborn stages, and a developmental decrease to approximately 30% α-Tpm phosphorylation in the adult mouse heart [28]. Interestingly, within the heart, there is differential Tpm phosphorylation among the four cardiac chambers, with atria exhibiting the highest level of phosphorylation ([30], and Sheikh and Wieczorek unpub. result). We have also found Tpm phosphorylation in human hearts; we determined Tpm is phosphorylated in substantial amounts in both the left and right ventricles, in addition to the interventricular septum. The amount of Tpm phosphorylation that occurs in human atria is currently unknown.

Several different kinases are implicated in the phosphorylation of striated muscle Tpm at the serine 283 amino acid. Investigators have identified tropomyosin kinase, protein kinase A, and protein kinase Cζ as playing potential roles in this process [15, 17, 31–33]. Also, a kinase isolated from chicken embryos has been found to phosphorylate Tpm [32]. Recent studies by our laboratory determined that casein kinase 2 can phosphorylate the striated muscle α-Tpm isoform, and this phosphorylation is specific for the S283 amino acid residue [29]. It is possible that dependent upon conditions (i.e., fetal vs. adult stages, skeletal vs. cardiac muscle, normal physiologic conditions vs. hypertrophic stress vs. physiological stress) that different kinases are activated to phosphorylate striated muscle Tpm in a myofiber-specific manner at different developmental stages and/or physiological conditions. Determining this relationship between specific kinases and their phosphorylation activity on Tpm is an area for future exploration.

3. Constitutive phosphorylation of Tpm leads to dilated cardiomyopathy

Previous investigations addressed the functional effect of phosphorylated Tpm using *in vitro* biochemical systems. As mentioned, biochemical assays, myofiber analyses, and molecular simulations indicate Tpm phosphorylation enhances the stiffness of the head-to-tail Tpm overlap region and its binding to TnT, while decreasing myofibril relaxation without significantly affecting cooperativity or altering activation kinetics [11, 22, 34]. Recently, we embarked on studies to address the physiological importance of Tpm phosphorylation in the heart using an *in vivo* model system [29]. The system we employed involved generating transgenic (TG) mice that expressed a phosphorylation mimetic specifically in the heart. Using the α-myosin heavy chain promoter (α-MHC), an α-Tpm cDNA construct that incorporated an aspartic acid residue replacement of serine at amino acid 283 (S283D) was expressed specifically in murine cardiomyocytes (**Figure 3**). Usage of an aspartic acid residue, which is negatively charged, mimics the negative charges found with phosphorylated amino acids, thus representing a pseudophosphorylation event.

Dilated cardiomyopathy (DCM) is a cause of significant morbidity and mortality in human patients. DCM is characterized by chamber dilation, systolic and/or diastolic dysfunction, arrhythmias, and sudden cardiac death. Results show that Tpm S283D mice that express high levels of the transgenic protein exhibit a severe dilated cardiomyopathy within 2 weeks postpartum (**Figure 4**). Similar to other Tpm transgenic mice, expression of the exogenous Tpm transgene leads to a reciprocal decrease in the endogenous Tpm protein, thereby demonstrating a translational feedback mechanism that regulates the total amount of Tpm protein in the cardiomyocytes [35]. This regulatory mechanism controlling Tpm protein levels is also operative when one allele of the Tpm gene is ablated [36]. In Tpm S283D mice, there is also a significant increase in the heart:body weight ratio, and these mice usually die by 1 month of age. A morphological and histological analysis of the Tpm S283D mice that express moderate levels of the transgene shows the hearts display a mild cardiomyocyte hypertrophy with limited fibrosis [29]. This moderate phenotype does not appear to progress to a more severe condition, even after 1 year. In addition, there are no significant differences in the heart:body weight ratio at either

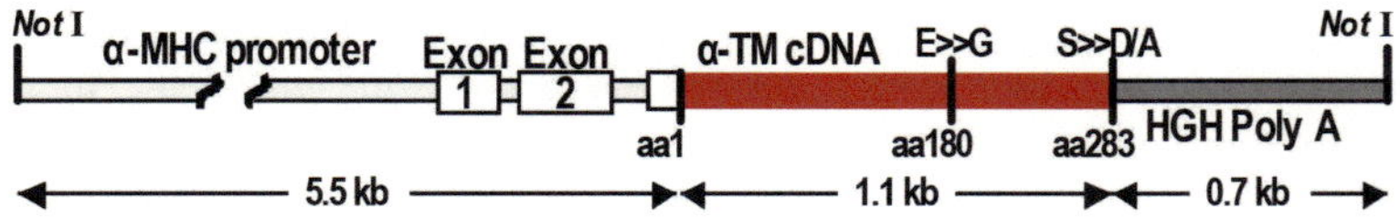

Figure 3.
Structure of a DNA transgenic construct showing the positions of the amino acid changes in the generation of Tpm mouse models. The striated muscle α-Tpm cDNA was ligated to the α-MHC promoter and the human growth hormone 3' UTR. Various changes in the Tpm amino acid sequences are indicated above the construct: the HCM mutation glutamic acid (E) is substituted for glycine (G); the phosphor-mimetic aspartic acid (D) is substituted for serine (S); the nonphosphorylatable alanine (A) is substituted for serine (S).

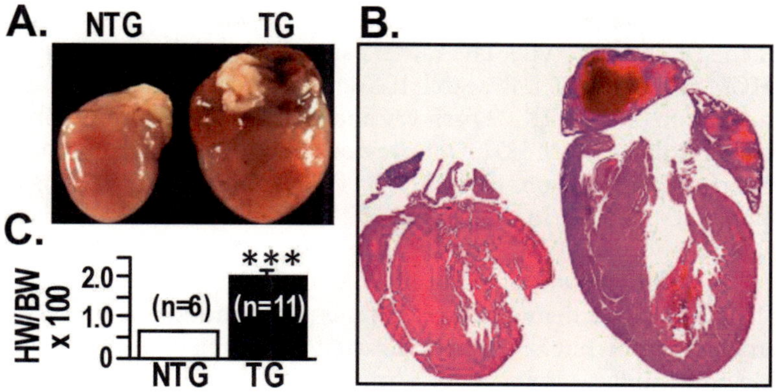

Figure 4.
*Control and Tpm S283D mouse hearts. A. Whole hearts of control (left) and TG (right). B. H & E staining of NTG (left) and TG (right) cross sections. C. Measurement of heart:body weight ratio. ***P < 0.0001 NTG vs. TG [29].*

3 or 6 months of age. Interestingly, these hearts do display significant physiological differences that are similar to those exhibited by dilated cardiomyopathic hearts.

To understand the functional significance of Tpm phosphorylation, we conducted various physiological measurements of cardiac and myofilament function. The work-performing heart model was used to obtain an *ex vivo* assessment of cardiac performance. Measurements were obtained to assess both contractile and relaxation parameters in the few high-expression mice that survived to 6 months of age, and in moderate expression mice; the results were similar regardless of the level of expression of the transgene. The values obtained show that there are no significant differences in the rates of contraction (+dP/dt) or in the time to peak pressure (TPP); however, the rates of relaxation (−dP/dt) is significantly reduced, concomitant with an increase in the half-time to relaxation (RT ½) (**Table 1**). Additional studies determined that the reduced relaxation performance by Tpm S283D hearts is maintained during maximal stimulation with isoproterenol, a β-adrenergic agonist that stimulates muscle contraction and relaxation. To determine whether the relationship between Ca^{2+} concentration and force-tension development is altered in myofibers at the sarcomeric level in Tpm S283D hearts with the phosphomimetic residue, we analyzed skinned fiber bundles from the papillary muscle of moderate and high-expression mice. No significant changes in absolute tension or normalized tension in NTG vs. TG mice are found (**Table 1**). Additionally, there are no significant differences in pCa_{50} or the Hill coefficient, a measure of the cooperative activation of the thin filament of the sarcomere.

Mouse model	Maximum rate of contraction	Maximum rate of relaxation	Myofiber Ca^{2+} sensitivity	Sarcomere tension development
α-Tpm	100%	100%	100%	100%
α-Tpm S283D	100%	↓	100%	100%
α-Tpm S283A	100%	100%	100%	100%
HCM α-Tpm E180G	100%	↓	↑	↑
HCM α-Tpm E180G/S283A	↑	100%	100%	100%

Table 1.
Physiological parameters of cardiac and myofiber function in Tpm mouse models.

We investigated potential signaling molecules that may play a role in the development of the DCM phenotype. The ERK1/2 signaling pathway regulates a balance between HCM and DCM [37]. Research has determined that there is a correlation between activation of the ERK1/2 pathway and HCM, whereas inhibition of the ERK pathway results in DCM [37]. Our previous investigations found that Tpm 54 DCM hearts have alterations in the levels of various kinases, including ERK1/2 and phosphor ERK1/2 [38]. In the Tpm S283D hearts, we find decreased expression of ERK1/2, phosphorylated ERK1/2, phosphorylated RSK3, and JNK1 which are members of the ERK pathway and associated with DCM. Thus, our current work on Tpm phosphorylation demonstrates that this posttranslational process not only affects cardiac function but also activates various signaling pathways associated with physiological and cardiomyopathic processes.

4. Tpm dephosphorylation leads to compensated cardiac hypertrophy

Although previous *in vitro* investigations addressed the effect of Tpm phosphorylation on myofilament function, studies have not examined the functional importance of Tpm dephosphorylation. To investigate the *in vivo* effect of decreased or ablated Tpm phosphorylation, we substituted serine 283 with an alanine (S283A), removing the phosphorylation site and effectively inhibiting the ability of α-Tpm to be phosphorylated. Transgenic mice were generated using the cardiac-specific myosin heavy chain promoter coupled to the α-Tpm S283A cDNA (**Figure 3**) [14]. Exogenous non-phosphorylatable Tpm protein expression ranged from 86 to 94%, with a concomitant reciprocal decrease in the endogenous Tpm levels. Interestingly, morphological analyses on these transgenic mouse hearts show only a very mild increase in cardiomyocyte disarray, along with a significant increase in cardiomyocyte area. Results also show no changes in the heart-to-body weight ratio, most likely due to the moderate nature of this hypertrophy. There are also no differences in the survival of these transgenic mice.

To address the functional significance of Tpm dephosphorylation, we employed myofilament calcium sensitivity assays, echocardiography, and the work-performing heart model. Skinned fiber bundles from adult papillary muscle TG mice show no significant changes in absolute tension or normalized tension from the Tpm S283A hearts (**Table 1**) [14]. Additionally, there are no significant differences in myofiber calcium sensitivity, pCa_{50} value, or the Hill coefficient. These results demonstrate that the relationship between Ca^{2+} concentration and force-tension development is similar in control and Tpm S283A myofilaments at the sarcomeric level. The work-performing heart model allows an *ex vivo* functional analysis of murine cardiac physiology. To determine the physiological effects of decreased Tpm phosphorylation in the Tpm S283A hearts, contractile and relaxation parameters were determined. Results showed that there are no changes in contractile and relaxation parameters in TG hearts, either under basal conditions or when isoproterenol is administered (**Table 1**) [14]. To assess whether decreased Tpm phosphorylation levels has an effect on *in vivo* cardiac function, we performed echocardiographic analysis. No physiological changes in heart function between control and TG mice as shown by fractional shorting, cardiac output, or ejection fraction are observed. However, there are sex-specific differences in cardiac morphology: male TG animals show significant increases in left ventricular mass and left ventricular anterior and posterior wall thickness, thus indicating a hypertrophic phenotype without associated functional defects. Female TG mice do not demonstrate any altered morphological or physiological effects in their hearts. Differences in the development of cardiac hypertrophy between sexes have been reported previously [39, 40] and demonstrate the moderate nature of this hypertrophic phenotype.

The lack of changes in cardiac function, myofilament cooperativity, and Ca^{2+} sensitivity, coupled with the development of compensated hypertrophy, lead to an investigation of possible signaling mechanisms involved in cardiac compensated or physiological hypertrophy. The Tpm S283A hearts exhibit no changes in common cardiomyopathic markers, such as β-myosin heavy chain, brain natriuretic peptide (BNP), and atrial natriuretic peptide (ANP) [14]. We did find that Tpm S283A hearts exhibit increased levels of SERCA2a protein. Total phospholamban protein expression is unchanged; however, phosphorylated phospholamban protein is increased. These alterations in Ca^{2+} handling proteins may be necessary to maintain normal cardiac function as the hearts compensate for the dephosphorylated Tpm that is incorporated into their myofilaments. Physiological cardiac hypertrophy is often associated with increased levels of SERCA2a, but without alterations in total phospholamban protein levels. Animals that exhibit physiological or compensated hypertrophy associated with exercise training appear to have cardiomyopathy marker and Ca^{2+} handling expression profiles that are similar to the Tpm S283A hearts, although the molecular expression profile during exercise training is not well elucidated. Collectively, our results demonstrate that Tpm dephosphorylation plays a role in the maintenance of a physiological or compensated hypertrophic phenotype. An area of future investigation would be to determine the level of Tpm phosphorylation in mouse hearts undergoing exercise training and exhibiting compensated cardiac hypertrophy.

5. Decreasing Tpm phosphorylation rescues hypertrophic cardiomyopathy

Mutations in cardiac contractile proteins are associated with the development of hypertrophic cardiomyopathy (HCM), also referred to familial hypertrophic cardiomyopathy (FHC). This disease is characterized by left and/or right ventricular hypertrophy, myocyte disarray, fibrosis, and cardiac arrhythmias that may lead to premature sudden death. At least 11 point mutations have been defined in Tpm that lead to HCM [41]. Work in our lab shows that the HCM Tpm mutation E180G in transgenic mice leads to a severe hypertrophic cardiomyopathy, similar to the phenotype exhibited by human patients [42, 43]. These TG mice exhibit significantly enlarged left ventricles, left and right atria, with disorganized myocytes and increased fibrosis. The hearts of these mice also exhibit physiological dysfunction, including decreased rates of relaxation, increased myofiber Ca^{2+} sensitivity, and increased maximum tension (**Table 1**) [43, 44]. Previous work in our laboratory found that mating these Tpm E180G mice with α-/β-Tpm chimeric mice could "rescue" double-transgenic progeny from the HCM phenotype [45]. This rescue from the severe physiological and pathological consequences of the HCM mutation was mediated by the attenuation of myofilament Ca^{2+} sensitivity by exchanging amino acids at the carboxy terminus from the α-Tpm to β-Tpm isoform, a region of Tpm that interacts with troponin T. This work demonstrated that alterations in the calcium response mediated through contractile proteins can prevent the pathological and physiological effects of HCM.

Our aforementioned investigations show that decreasing Tpm phosphorylation can lead to a compensated hypertrophic phenotype with significant increases in SERCA2a expression and phosphorylation of phospholamban. Since we determined that cardiac hypertrophy could be phenotypically rescued through modification of the response of the myocyte to Ca^{2+}, we decided to further test this hypothesis. We generated TG mice that coexpressed the HCM α-Tpm E180G mutation with the α-Tpm S283A mutation in the same expression construct [27]. These double mutant transgenic (DMTG) mouse hearts express 50–64% exogenous Tpm protein, coupled with a concomitant decrease in endogenous Tpm protein; the amount of

Tpm phosphorylation in these double TG mice was minimal, similar to the levels found in the Tpm S283A mouse hearts. A detailed histological and morphological analysis show that the DMTG hearts exhibit a phenotype that is very similar to age-matched control mice with no cardiomyocyte disarray, atrial or ventricular enlargement, or excessive fibrosis, changes which are characteristic of the Tpm E180G hearts (**Figure 5**) [27]. Also, there were no differences in heart weight:body weight ratios between control and DMTG animals. The addition of the S283A amino acid substitution into the HCM α-Tpm E180G mice considerably extended the life expectancy of these DMTG mice to that of wild-type control mice.

To determine whether decreased Tpm phosphorylation could improve cardiac function in a model of hypertrophic cardiomyopathy, we performed echocardiography on the DMTG mouse hearts and force-Ca^{2+} measurements on skinned papillary muscle fiber bundles. Results show improved systolic function with increases in ejection fraction and fractional shortening when compared with α-Tpm E180G and control littermates (**Table 1**) [27]. In addition, diastolic function is significantly improved in the DMTG animals, which demonstrates the rescue from the extreme diastolic dysfunction seen in the HCM α-Tpm E180G mice. We measured myofilament Ca^{2+} sensitivity in the DMTG mice to determine whether this parameter could also contribute to the improved cardiac function. Myofilaments from the DMTG mice show a significant decrease in Ca^{2+} sensitivity when compared with the HCM α-Tpm E180G measurements as indicated by a lower pCa_{50} value; the maximum tension and Hill coefficient are not significantly different among control, HCM α-Tpm E180G, and DMTG myofilaments. The conclusion of these results demonstrates that decreased phosphorylation of Tpm can morphologically and physiologically rescue the pathological phenotype associated with HCM.

To examine potential signaling mechanisms that may be operative in DMTG animals that might play a role in the rescue of the HCM phenotype, we assayed gene expression of cardiomyopathy markers and Ca^{2+}-handling proteins. Results show that β-myosin heavy chain (β-MHC), BNP, and ANP exhibit significantly lower levels than those found in the HCM α-Tpm E180G hearts; the levels in the DMTG animals are similar to control mice [27]. Results show there are no differences in SERCA2a levels among control, α-Tpm E180G, and DMTG animals, but there is an increase in total PLN phosphorylation in the DMTG mice. It is possible that this

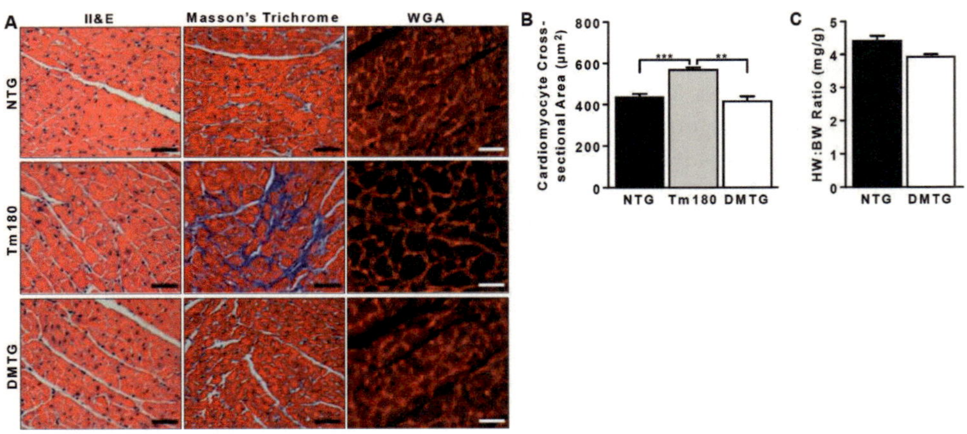

Figure 5.
A. Histological studies of NTG, Tm180, and DMTG hearts at 3 months of age stained with H&E, Masson's trichrome, and wheat germ agglutinin (WGA). Images were taken at 40×, and scale bars indicate 50 μm. B. Cardiomyocyte cross-sectional area measurements (n = 6). C. Heart weight-to-body weight (HW:BW) ratios at 3 months of age (n = 6). Error bars represent S.E. [27].

increase in PLN phosphorylation releases the inhibition on SERCA2a, thus stimulating Ca^{2+} resequestration into the sarcoplasmic reticulum to help rescue the HCM phenotype in the DMTG hearts. Other studies show that modification in contractile protein phosphorylation can improve sarcomeric and cardiac function. Deletion of the amino-terminal cardiac troponin I (TnI) domain improves cardiac contractility in aged mice, and cardiac function can be improved in restrictive cardiomyopathy mice when crossed with a TG mouse expressing a truncated amino-terminal TnI molecule [46, 47]. Also, phosphorylation of myosin light chain kinase can normalize increased Ca^{2+} sensitivity in an HCM model of regulatory light chain [48]. The molecular mechanism(s) that is activated by decreasing Tpm phosphorylation to improve cardiac function is unknown; however, studies suggest that the MEK1-ERK1/2 pathway may be involved in reversing the α-Tpm E180G hypertrophy [49, 50]. Another signaling pathway that might be involved in preventing the disease phenotype in the DMTG mice involves protein phosphatase 2a and casein-kinse-2-interacting protein (CKIP-1). The HCM Tpm E180G mice have increased levels of PP2a and casein kinase-2 [51, 52]. CKIP-1 and PP2a directly interact [53], which facilitates the binding of PP2a to HDAC4 to promote HDAC's dephosphorylation. Dephosphorylation of HDAC suppresses cardiac hypertrophy and the fetal cardiac gene program [53]. If decreased Tpm phosphorylation leads to increased levels of CKIP-1 expression, then this signaling pathway may be activated in the rescue DMTG mice.

6. Conclusions

As cited above, these studies collectively demonstrate a significant biological and physiological role for Tpm phosphorylation under both normal and cardiomyopathic conditions. The penultimate Tpm amino acid, serine residue 283, is located in a carboxyl region that is associated with multiple protein interactions: dimers between C-terminal Tpm molecules, C-terminal Tpm overlapping with N-terminal Tpm, and C-terminal Tpm binding with N-terminal troponin T. These multiple protein-protein interacting regions regulate myofilament function and cardiac performance, and are dramatically altered with changes in Tpm phosphorylation. Understanding the significance of developmental and disease associated changes that occur in Tpm phosphorylation is an area for future exploration. In addition, determining whether changes in Tpm phosphorylation are causative or a consequence of HCM is vital to developing therapeutic strategies for cardiovascular disease. An area of future investigation is to identify drug targets for the various kinases that phosphorylate Tpm and their downstream signaling factors so as to potentially treat various cardiomyopathic conditions.

Acknowledgements

The author wishes to acknowledge the invaluable contributions of the many investigators and collaborators of the work presented in this article, especially Drs. E. Schulz, S. Rajan, and G. Jagatheesan.

Conflict of interest

There are no conflicts of interest to report.

Author details

David F. Wieczorek
University of Cincinnati College of Medicine, Cincinnati, Ohio, USA

*Address all correspondence to: david.wieczorek@uc.edu

References

[1] Wieczorek D, Smith C, Nadal-Ginard B. The rat α-tropomyosin gene generates minimum of six different mRNAs coding for striated, smooth and nonmuscle isoforms by alternative splicing. Molecular and Cellular Biology. 1988;**8**:679-694

[2] Vrhovski B, Theze N, Thiebaud P. Structure and evolution of tropomyosin genes. In: Gunning P, editor. Tropomyosin. Austin, Texas, USA: Landes Bioscience; 2008. pp. 6-26

[3] Cummins P, Perry S. Chemical and immunochemical characteristics of tropomyosins from striated and smooth muscle. The Biochemical Journal. 1974;**141**:43-49

[4] Izumo S, Nadal-Ginard B, Mahdavi V. Protooncogene induction and reprogramming of cardiac gene expression produced by pressure overload. Proceedings of the National Academy of Sciences of the United States of America. 1988;**85**:339-343

[5] Muthuchamy M, Pajak L, Howles P, Doetschman T, Wieczorek DF. Developmental analysis of tropomyosin gene expression in embryonic stem cells and mouse embryos. Molecular and Cellular Biology. 1993;**13**:3311-3323

[6] Rajan S, Jagatheesan G, Karam C, Alves M, Bodi I, Schwartz A, et al. Molecular and functional characterization of a novel cardiac specific human tropomyosin isoform. Circulation. 2010;**121**:410-418

[7] Denz C, Narshi A, Zajdel R, Dube D. Expression of a novel cardiac-specific tropomyosin isoform in humans. Biochemical and Biophysical Research Communications. 2004;**320**:1291-1297

[8] Yuan C, Sheng Q, Tang H, Li Y, Zeng R, Solaro RJ. Quantitative comparison of sarcomeric phosphoproteomes of neonatal and adult rat hearts. American Journal of Physiology. Heart and Circulatory Physiology. 2008;**295**:H647-H656

[9] Sadayappan S, Osinska H, Klevitsky R, Lorenz J, Sargent M, Molkentin J, et al. Cardiac myosin binding protein C phosphorylation is cardioprotective. Proceedings of the National Academy of Sciences of the United States of America. 2006;**103**:16918-16923

[10] Moss R, Fitzsimons D. Myosin light chain 2 into the mainstream of cardiac development and contractility. Circulation Research. 2006;**99**:225-227

[11] Lu Q, Hinken A, Patrick S, Solaro RJ, Kobayashi T. Phosphorylation of cardiac troponin I at protein kinase C site threonine 144 depresses cooperative activation of thin filaments. The Journal of Biological Chemistry. 2010;**285**:11810-11817

[12] van der Velden J, Narolska N, Lamberts R, Boontje N, Borbely A, Zaremba R, et al. Functional effects of protein kinase C-mediated myofilament phosphorylation in human myocardium. Cardiovascular Research. 2006;**69**:876-887

[13] Heeley D, Moir A, Perry S. Phosphorylation of tropomyosin during development in mammalian striated muscle. FEBS Letters. 1982;**146**:115-118

[14] Schulz E, Correll R, Sheikh H, Lofrano-Alves M, Engel P, Newman G, et al. Tropomyosin dephosphorylation results in compensated cardiac hypertrophy. The Journal of Biological Chemistry. 2012;**287**:44478-44489

[15] Heeley D, Watson M, Mak A, Dubord P, Smillie L. Effect of phosphorylation on the interaction and functional properties of rabbit

striated muscle αα-tropomyosin. The Journal of Biological Chemistry. 1989;**264**:2424-2430

[16] Heeley D. Investigation of the effects of phosphorylation of rabbit striated muscle αα-tropomyosin and rabbit skeletal muscle troponin-T. European Journal of Biochemistry. 1994;**221**: 129-137

[17] Mak A, Smillie L, Barany M. Specific phosphorylation at serine-283 of α-tropomyosin from frog skeletal and rabbit skeletal and cardiac muscle. Proceedings of the National Academy of Sciences of the United States of America. 1978;**75**:3588-3592

[18] Greenfield N, Huang Y, Swapna G, Bhattacharya A, Rapp B, Singh A, et al. Solution NMR structure of the junction between tropomyosin molecules: Implications for actin binding and regulation. Journal of Molecular Biology. 2006;**364**:80-96

[19] Butters C, Willadsen K, Tobacman L. Cooperative interactions between adjacent troponin-tropomyosin complexes may be transmitted through the actin filament. The Journal of Biological Chemistry. 1993;**268**:15565-15570

[20] Dabrowska R, Nowak E, Drabikowski W. Some functional properties of nonpolymerizable and polymerizable tropomyosin. Journal of Muscle Research and Cell Motility. 1983;**4**:143-161

[21] Walsh T, Trueblood C, Evans R, Weber A. Removal of tropomyosin overlap and the co-operative response to increasing calcium concentrations of the acto-subfragment −1 ATPase. Journal of Molecular Biology. 1984;**182**:265-269

[22] Nixon B, Liu B, Scellini B, Tesi C, Piroddi N, Ogut O, et al. Tropomyosin Ser-283 pseudo-phosphorylation slows myofibril relaxation. Archives of Biochemistry and Biophysics. 2013;**535**:30-38

[23] Rao V, Clobes A, Guilford W. Force spectroscopy reveals multiple "closed states" of the muscle thin filament. The Journal of Biological Chemistry. 2011;**286**:24135-24141

[24] Lehrer S, Morris E. Dual effects of tropomyhosin and troponin-tropomyosin on actomyosin subfragment 1 ATPase. The Journal of Biological Chemistry. 1982;**257**:807308080

[25] Lehrer S, Geeves M. The muscle thin filament as a classical cooperative/ allosteric regulatory system. Journal of Molecular Biology. 1998;**277**: 1081-1089

[26] Jagatheesan G, Rajan S, Petrashevska N, Schwartz A, Boivin G, Vahebi S, et al. Functional importance of the carboxyl-terminal region of striated muscle tropomyosin. The Journal of Biological Chemistry. 2003;**278**:23204-23211

[27] Schulz E, Wilder T, Chowdhury S, Sheikh H, Wolska B, Solaro RJ, et al. Decreasing tropomyosin phosphorylation rescues tropomyosin-induced familial hypertrophic cardiomyopathy. The Journal of Biological Chemistry. 2013;**288**:28925-28935

[28] Schulz E, Wieczorek DF. Tropomyosin de-phosphorylation in the heart: What are the consequences? Journal of Muscle Research and Cell Motility. 2013;**34**:239-246

[29] Rajan S, Jagatheesan G, Petrashevskaya N, Biesiadecki B, Warren C, Riddle T, Liggett S, Wolska B, Solaro RJ, Wieczorek DF. Tropomyosin Pseudo-Phosphorylation Results in Dilated Cardiomyopathy. The Journal of Biological Chemistry. In revision.

[30] Heeley D. Phosphorylation of tropomyosin in striated muscle. Journal of Muscle Research and Cell Motility. 2014;**24**:233-237

[31] Reddy Y, Ballard D, Giri N, Schwartz A. Phosphorylation of cardiac native tropomyosin and troponin. Inhibitory effect of actomyosin and possible presence of endogenous myofibrillar-located cyclic-AMP-dependent protein kinase. Journal of Molecular and Cellular Cardiology. 1973;**5**:461-471

[32] Montgomery K, Mak A. *In vitro* phosphorylation of tropomyosin by a kinase from chicken embryo. The Journal of Biological Chemistry. 1984;**259**:5555-5560

[33] Wu S, Solaro RJ. Protein kinase Cζ. A novel regulator of both phosphorylation and dephosphorylation of cardiac sarcomeric proteins. The Journal of Biological Chemistry. 2007;**282**:30691-30698

[34] Lehman W, Medlock G, Li X, Suphamungmee W, Tu A, Schmidtmann A, et al. Phosphorylation of Ser283 enhances the stiffness of the tropomyosin head-to-tail overlap domain. Archives of Biochemistry and Biophysics. 2015;**571**:10-15

[35] Muthuchamy M, Grupp I, Grupp G, O'Toole B, Kier A, Boivin G, et al. Molecular and physiological effects of overexpressing striated muscle β-tropomyosin in the adult murine heart. The Journal of Biological Chemistry. 1995;**270**:30593-30603

[36] Rethinasamy P, Muthuchamy M, Boivin G, Wolska B, Evans C, Solaro RJ, et al. Molecular and physiological effects of α-tropomyosin ablation in the mouse. Circulation Research. 1998;**82**: 116-123

[37] Kehat I, Davis J, Tiburcy M, Accornero F, Saba-El-Leil M, Maillet M, et al. Extracellular signal-regulated kinases 1 and 2 regulate the balance between eccentric and concentric cardiac growth. Circulation Research. 2011;**108**:176-183

[38] Alves M, Warren C, Simon J, Gaffin R, Montminy E, Wieczorek DF, et al. Early sensitization of myofilaments of Ca^{2+} prevents genetically linked dilated cardiomyopathy in mice. Cardiovascular Research. 2017;**113**:915-925

[39] Donaldson C, Eder S, Baker C, Aronovitz M, Weiss A, Hall-Porter M, et al. Estrogen attenuates left ventricular and cardiomyocyte hypertrophy by an estrogen receptor-dependent pathway that increases calcineurin degradation. Circulation Research. 2009;**104**:265-275

[40] Gardner J, Brower G, Woloshenyuk T, Janicki J. Cardioprotectioin in female rats subjected to chronic volume overload. Synergistic interaction of estrogen and phytoestrogens. American Journal of Physiology. Heart and Circulatory Physiology. 2008;**294**:H198-H204

[41] Wieczorek DF, Jagatheesan G, Sudarsan R. The role of tropomyosin in heart disease. In: Gunning P, editor. Tropomyosin. Landes Bioscience; 2008. pp. 132-142

[42] Thierfelder L, Watkins H, MacRae C, Lamas R, McKenna W, Vosberg H, et al. α-Tropomyosin and cardiac troponin T mutations cause familial hypertrophic cardiomyopathy: A disease of the sarcomere. Cell. 1994;**77**:701-712

[43] Prabhakar R, Boivin G, Grupp I, Hoit B, Arteaga G, Solaro RJ, et al. A familial hypertrophic cardiomyopathy α-tropomyosin mutation causes severe cardiac hypertrophy and death in mice. Journal of Molecular and Cellular Cardiology. 2001;**33**:1815-1828

[44] Prabhakar R, Petrashevskaya N, Schwartz A, Aronow B, Boivin G,

Molkentin J, et al. A mouse model of familial hypertrophic cardiomyopathy caused by a α-tropomyosin mutation. Molecular and Cellular Biochemistry. 2001;**251**:33-42

[45] Jagatheesan G, Rajan S, Petrashevska N, Schwartz A, Boivin G, Arteaga G, et al. Rescue of familial hypertrophic cardiomyopathy mice by desensitizing myofilament calcium response. American Journal of Physiology-Heart and Circulatory Physiology. 2007;**293**:H949-H958

[46] Biesiadecki B, Tachampa K, Yuan C, Jin J, de Tombe P, Solaro RJ. Removal of the cardiac troponin 1 N-terminal extensioin improves cardiac function in aged mice. The Journal of Biological Chemistry. 2010;**285**:19688-19698

[47] Li Y, Charles P, Nan C, Pinto J, Wang Y, Liang J, et al. Correcting diastolic dysfunction by Ca^{2+} desensitizing troponin in a transgenic mouse model of restrictive cardiomyopathy. Journal of Molecular and Cellular Cardiology. 2010;**49**:402-411

[48] Muthu P, Kazmierczak K, Jones M, Szczesna-Cordary D. The effect of myosin RLC phosphorylation in normal and cardiomyopathic mouse hearts. Journal of Cellular and Molecular Medicine. 2012;**16**:911-919

[49] Gaffin R, Pena J, Alves M, Dias F, Chowdhury S, Heinrich L, et al. Long-term rescue of a familial hypertrophic cardiomyopathy caused by a mutation in the thin filament protein, tropomyosin, via modulation of a calcium cycling protein. Journal of Molecular and Cellular Cardiology. 2011;**51**:812-820

[50] Bueno O, De Windt L, Tymitz K, Witt S, Kimball T, Klevitsky R, et al. The MEK1-ERK1/2 signaling pathway promotes compensate cardiac hypertrophy in transgenic mice. The EMBO Journal. 2000;**19**:6341-6350

[51] Al Moamen N, Prasad V, Bodi I, Miller M, Neiman M, Lasko V, et al. Loss of the AE3 anion exchanger in a hypertrophic cardiomyopathy model causes rapid decompensation and heart failure. Journal of Molecular and Cellular Cardiology. 2011;**50**:137-146

[52] Rajan S, Sheikh H, Schulz E, Jagatheesan G, Wieczorek DF. Regulation of Tropomyosin Phosphorylation in Normal and Cardiomyopathic Hearts. American Heart Association; 2010; Abstr. 17a

[53] Ling S, Sun Q, Li Y, Zhang L, Zhang P, Wang X, et al. CKIP-1 inhibits cardiac hypertrophy by regulating class 11 histone deacetylase phosphorylation through recruiting PP2a. Circulation. 2012;**126**:3028-3040

Chapter 3

Waveform Capnography for Monitoring Ventilation during Cardiopulmonary Resuscitation: The Problem of Chest Compression Artifact

Mikel Leturiondo, Sofía Ruiz de Gauna, José Julio Gutiérrez, Digna M. González-Otero, Jesus M. Ruiz, Luis A. Leturiondo and Purificación Saiz

Abstract

Sudden cardiac arrest (SCA) is the sudden cessation of the heart's effective pumping function, confirmed by the absence of pulse and breathing. Without appropriate treatment, it leads to sudden cardiac death, considered responsible for half of the global cardiac disease deaths. Cardiopulmonary resuscitation (CPR) is a key intervention during SCA. Current resuscitation guidelines emphasize the use of waveform capnography during CPR in order to enhance CPR quality and improve patient outcomes. Capnography represents the concentration of the partial pressure of carbon dioxide (CO_2) in respiratory gases and reflects ventilation and perfusion of the patient. Waveform capnography should be used for confirming the correct placement of the tracheal tube and monitoring ventilation. Other potential uses of capnography in resuscitation involve monitoring CPR quality, early identification of restoration of spontaneous circulation (ROSC), and determination of patient prognosis. An important role of waveform capnography is ventilation rate monitoring to prevent overventilation. However, some studies have reported the appearance of high-frequency oscillations synchronized with chest compressions superimposed on the capnogram. This chapter explores the incidence of chest compression artifact in out-of-hospital capnograms, assesses its negative influence in the automated detection of ventilations, and proposes several methods to enhance ventilation detection and capnography waveform.

Keywords: cardiopulmonary resuscitation, advanced life support, waveform capnography, ventilation, chest compression artifact

1. Introduction

In the past century, cardiac disease was declared as one of the leading causes of global death, comprising a 30% of the global mortality [1]. It is estimated that sudden cardiac death is responsible for half of all cardiac disease deaths [1, 2], affecting more than 300,000 victims per year in the United States and around 275,000 in the Europe [3–5]. About 80% of sudden cardiac deaths are caused by out-of-hospital cardiac arrests (OHCA) [1], defined as the sudden cessation of the heart's effective pumping function confirmed by the absence of pulse and breathing and occurring in an out-of-hospital setting [6].

During OHCA, there are two prehospital life supporting emergency medical services (EMS): basic life support (BLS) and advanced life support (ALS). BLS treatment is provided by emergency medical technicians and includes early CPR and early defibrillation, usually delivered with an automated external defibrillator (AED). ALS treatment procured by clinicians during CPR usually includes manual defibrillation, advanced airway placement, and drug administration, together with CPR [7, 8].

Several studies have reported a strong correlation between the quality of CPR and the chance of successful defibrillation [9–11]. Thus, resuscitation guidelines [12, 13] globally recommend providing chest compressions with a rate in the range of 100 and 120 compressions per minute (cpm) and achieving a depth between 5 and 6 cm. Ventilations should be provided with a 30 compressions-to-2 ventilations ratio before intubation. After intubation, ALS guidelines recommend continuous chest compressions and ventilations with a ventilation rate around 10 breaths per minute [7, 8]. Despite the fact that some studies have declared hyperventilation as harmful for patient outcome, by either high rate or volume [14, 15], excessive ventilation rates (as high as 30 breaths per minute) are common in resuscitation [16–18]. Many animal studies revealed that high ventilation rates increased intrathoracic pressures and decreased coronary perfusion and survival rates [16, 19, 20]. However, another recent animal study reported no adverse hemodynamic effects, although they did observe a decrease in maximum CO_2 values [21].

In order to alleviate this problem and prevent inadvertent hyperventilation, resuscitation guidelines highlight the role of capnography for ventilation rate monitoring during CPR [7, 8]. Other advantages of capnography include assessment of the correct placement of the endotracheal tube [21], monitoring the quality of chest compressions [22], early identification of restoration of spontaneous circulation (ROSC) [23], and determination of patient prognosis [7, 24, 25].

This chapter analyzes the use of capnometry for ventilation monitoring during OHCA episodes. First, we briefly introduce the evolution of capnometry and the different technologies used in the field. Then, we characterize the capnography signal during ongoing CPR. The main conclusion of this analysis is that the appearance of high-frequency oscillations superimposed on the waveform capnography is frequent during resuscitation. We then analyze the impact of these oscillations on out-of-hospital automated detection of ventilations. Finally, we propose two methods to improve ventilation detection during CPR by filtering the artifact from the capnography signal and a method to enhance capnography waveform in the presence of artifact.

2. Evolution of capnometry

Since 1943, capnometry has become an essential component of standard anesthesia monitoring [26]. Capnometry represents the numerical value of the carbon dioxide (CO_2) partial pressure measurement in exhaled respiratory gases. The maximum CO_2 concentration at the end of the exhalation, known as end-tidal CO_2 ($ETCO_2$), reflects cardiac output and pulmonary blood flow. Preventing hypoxia, i.e., deprivation of adequate oxygen supply, during anesthesia is the primary goal of anesthesiologists. Improvements with capnometry in this field currently allow the early identification of harmful situations before hypoxia leads to irreversible brain damage. Because of these improvements, the use of capnography has spread from the operating room into emergency medicine environment and even into out-of-hospital emergency settings.

Several methods have been used to determine the presence and concentration of CO_2 over the years. The simplest form of CO_2 detection available is colorimetric capnometry. This technology is based on a paper that changes in color in the presence of CO_2, but its inability to detect breath-to-breath changes prohibits the use of this device to guide ventilation. Later, semiquantitative capnometers (**Figure 1a**) that provide a rough estimation of the $ETCO_2$ concentration have been developed. The technology behind these devices reports the $ETCO_2$ value in a series of stacked colors rather than providing a numerical value, being useful to confirm correct airway placement.

More recently, quantitative capnometry involving infrared spectrophotometric analysis of expired gases (**Figure 1b**) has led to the most accurate method to measure $ETCO_2$ values. This technology provides an end-tidal value for each breath, allowing an optimal control of ventilation. Improvements in the field allowed the graphical representation and recording of the CO_2 concentration throughout the breath (i.e., waveform capnography, **Figure 1c**).

Two different methods of gas sampling, illustrated in **Figure 2**, are used to measure quantitative capnometry and waveform capnography: mainstream and sidestream. The main difference is that mainstream is directly placed in the main flow of exhaled gases, while in sidestream little samples are aspirated with a capillary sampling tube. During the last two decades, improvements in high-flow sidestream capnometers turned into Microstream™ capnometers, with an aspiration flow rate of 50 ml min^{-1}. This technology uses a highly CO_2-specific infrared source where

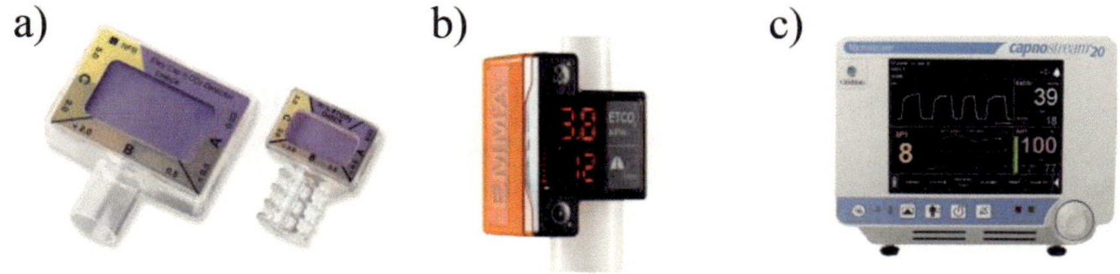

Figure 1.
Evolution of capnometry in out-of-hospital emergency settings. (a) Semiquantitative capnometer, (b) quantitative capnometer, and (c) waveform capnography. Courtesy of Medtronic and Masimo.

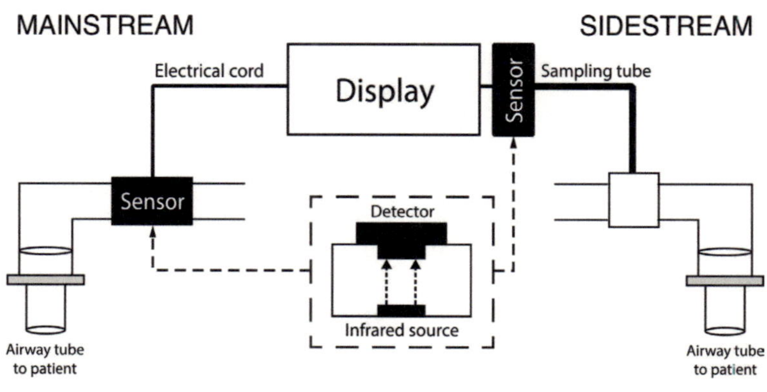

Figure 2.
Brief schemes of quantitative capnometry to acquire the capnography signal, mainstream and sidestream.

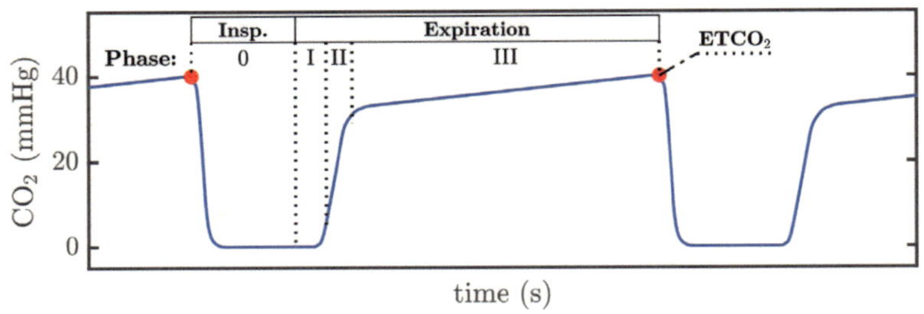

Figure 3.
The normal capnogram. Capnography waveform representing the variation of CO_2 concentration during the respiratory cycle. Segments and phases follow the nomenclature proposed by Bhavani-Shankar and Philip [27].

the IR emitter exactly matches the absorption spectrum of the CO_2 molecules. This facilitates the sample cell to use a much smaller volume that permits a low flow rate, being less likely to aspirate water and secretions.

The evolution and morphology of CO_2 concentration in the respiratory cycle of a normal capnogram are depicted in **Figure 3**. The initial rapid decrease of CO_2 concentration named as phase 0 represents the inspiration segment, where the lungs are filled with CO_2-free respiratory gases until a zero level is reached, defining the baseline of the capnogram. The following phases represent the expiration segment: during phase I, the CO_2-free gas in the anatomical dead space (between the alveoli and measurement device) is exhaled; in phase II a mixture of gases from the anatomical dead space and the alveoli quickly rises the level of CO_2 concentration; finally in phase III, CO_2-rich gases coming from the alveoli slowly raise the CO_2 concentration until a peak level is reached, corresponding to the $ETCO_2$ value [28].

3. Capnography signal during ongoing chest compressions

The initial use of capnographs during resuscitation was initially proposed by the International Liaison Committee on Resuscitation (ILCOR) in 2010, and since 2015 it is becoming a standard of care in advanced high-quality CPR [24, 29, 30]. Among the several advantages of waveform capnography during CPR emphasized in current resuscitation guidelines, but one of its most important roles is to monitor ventilation rate, helping to avoid overventilation.

For a reliable clinical analysis, either visual or automated, of the waveform capnography, its morphology is essential. All phases of the respiratory cycle must by identifiable during CPR, and the measurement of $ETCO_2$ should be possible. However, issues related to the capnograph as well as to the ongoing resuscitation efforts may distort the waveform capnography [29, 31, 32]. Moreover, the appearance of fast oscillations induced in the waveform capnography at different rates and with varying amplitude has been reported in several studies [33–35], often completely distorting the real tracing of the respiratory cycle as shown in **Figure 4b**.

To the best of our knowledge, studies assessing the incidence and origin of this artifact are sparse. A preliminary abstract published by Idris et al. [33] in 2010 analyzed a dataset of 210 patients and detected the presence of this artifact in 154 episodes, reporting an incidence greater than 70%. Several studies found that provided chest compressions generate passive ventilations of low inspiratory tidal volumes [33–35]. Deakin et al. [34] found that generated low tidal volumes during ongoing chest compressions were considerably lower than the anatomical dead space (150 ml). Recently, Vanwulpen et al. [35] conducted a similar out-of-hospital study, and their results were in line with the ones reported by Deakin et al., but they found lower inspiratory volumes. Therefore generated gas exchange is insufficient to properly ventilate the patient [36].

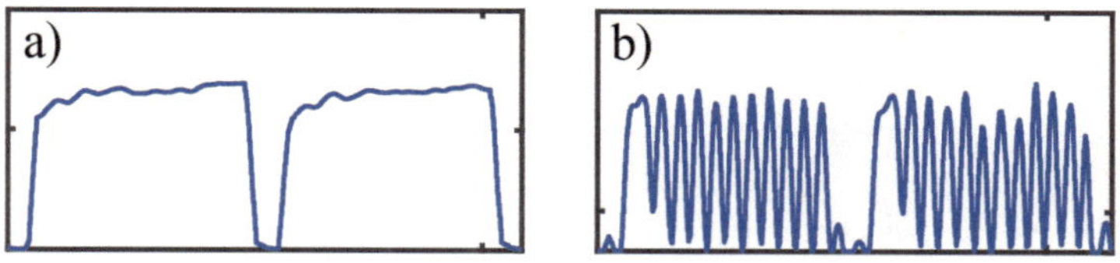

Figure 4.
OHCA waveform capnography signal segments. (a) Nondistorted waveform and (b) capnogram distorted by fast oscillations.

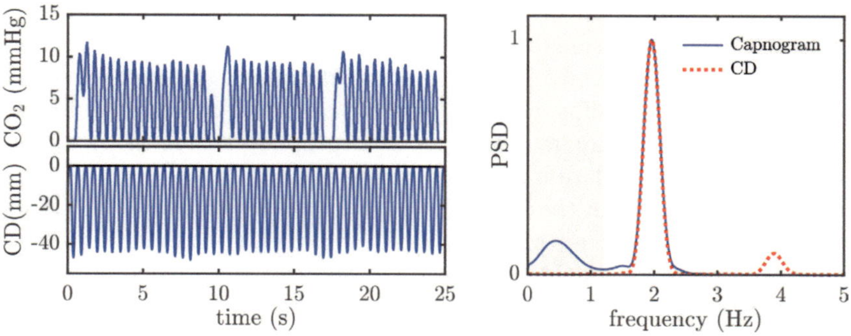

Figure 5.
Time-domain and spectral analyses of the oscillations present in a capnogram segment (top left). CD signal (bottom left). Normalized PSD analysis (right) of the distorted capnogram (solid blue) and of the CD signal (dotted red). The high-frequency peak around 2 Hz matches the average chest compression rate of 116 compressions per minute.

Our first approach was to assess the origin of the artifact, so we performed time-domain and spectral analyses on a large set of out-of-hospital capnograms. Readers are encouraged to consult reference [37] for further details. As an example, **Figure 5** depicts a distorted capnogram interval (top-left panel), the concurrent chest compression depth (CD) signal (bottom-left panel), and the normalized power spectral density (PSD) estimated (right panel) for both the waveform capnography signal (solid blue) and for the CD signal (dotted red). The PSD analysis of the waveform capnography reveals a low-frequency peak that represents the ventilation rate (shadowed in gray) and a high-frequency peak corresponding to the artifact oscillation frequency. The latter exactly overlaps with the fundamental frequency peak of the CD signal. Thus, the induced artifact presents a sinusoidal pattern with a fundamental frequency that matches the frequency of the chest compressions.

The appearance of the artifact induced by chest compressions can negatively affect the quality of CPR in three different aspects: first, causing misdetection of ventilations and consequently giving an incorrect feedback in the estimation of ventilation rate; second, impeding reliable and stable $ETCO_2$ measurements as reported by Raimondi et al. [38]; and third, interfering with CPR providers' waveform capnography interpretation.

4. Impact of chest compression artifact on ventilation detection

This section briefly describes the conducted analysis to characterize the morphology of the chest compression-induced oscillations and assess its impact on automated ventilation detection during ongoing CPR. First, we describe the process followed to collect the OHCA episodes used in the study, as well as the steps followed to annotate each ventilation instance. Then, we describe an algorithm designed to automatically detect ventilations in the capnogram. Finally, we assess the impact of the artifact on the reliability of ventilation detection by testing the performance of the detection algorithm. For a more detailed description of the database used and the methods followed, see Ref. [37].

4.1 Data collection and annotation

In order to perform the analysis, a dataset of 301 episodes was selected from a large database collected between 2011 and 2016 as part of the Resuscitation Outcomes Consortium (ROC), collected by the Portland Regional Clinical Centre (Oregon, USA). The data collection was approved by the Oregon Health and Science University (OHSU) Institutional Review Board (IRB00001736). No patient private data was required for this study. Episodes were recorded using Heartstart MRx monitor-defibrillators (Philips, USA), equipped with real-time CPR feedback technology (Q-CPR) and sidestream waveform capnography (Microstream, Oridion Systems Ltd., Israel). Ventilation was provided with a bag valve mask (BVM), endotracheal tube (ETT), or the King LT-D supraglottic airway (SGA).

Three biomedical engineers participating in the study visually reviewed and manually annotated each OHCA episode. Episodes were classified as distorted if evident chest compression-induced oscillations were found during more than 1 min of the total chest compression time. In the case of distorted episodes, experts annotated the location of the artifact with respect to the capnogram segment to characterize its morphology. Otherwise, episodes were grouped as nondistorted. Episodes and intervals with unreliable data caused by excessive noise or disconnections were discarded.

Figure 6 shows an example of the ventilation annotation process. The compression depth (CD) signal (top panel) was used to determine whether chest compressions were provided or not. The position of each single ventilation was also annotated using the TI signal as a reference. Provided ventilations provoke slow fluctuations in the TI signal [39–41]. The raw TI signal was low-pass filtered to enhance the slow fluctuations caused by ventilations (middle panel, blue line). Each ventilation was annotated at the instant corresponding to a rise in each impedance

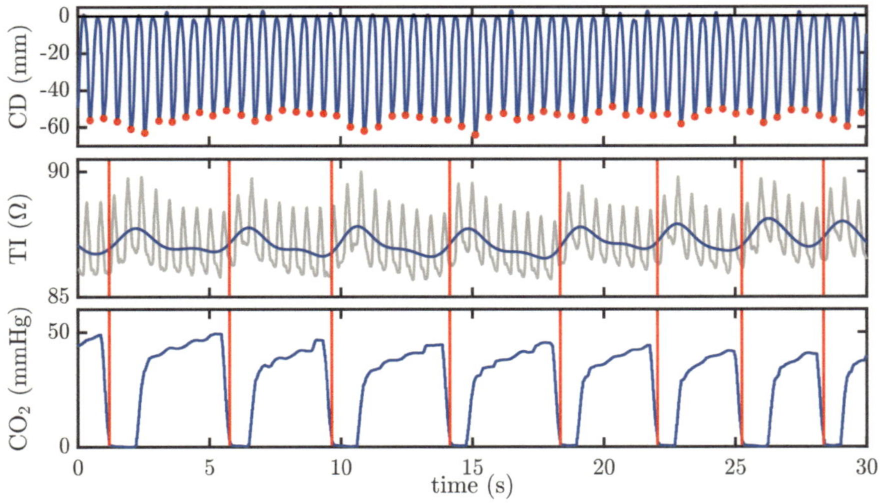

Figure 6.
CD signal measured with Q-CPR technology (top panel), raw TI signal acquired through defibrillation pads (middle panel, gray line) and waveform capnography (bottom panel). Using the low-pass filtered TI signal (middle panel, blue line), ventilations were annotated at the rise of a TI fluctuation, corresponding with a CO_2 rapid decay to zero.

fluctuation (vertical red line). The capnogram depicted in the bottom panel allows visual confirmation of the presence of ventilations. Resulting annotations were used as the gold standard to evaluate the performance of an automated capnogram-based ventilation detection algorithm.

4.2 Method for an automated capnogram-based ventilation detection

There is remarkably little knowledge about how the proprietary algorithm of a commercial capnometer works. In 2010, Edelson et al. [41] proposed the first algorithm to automatically detect ventilations in the capnogram during CPR. For this study, we designed a new algorithm for ventilation detection, based upon certain assumptions about the nature of the CO_2 waveform.

A simplified scheme of the algorithm performance is shown in **Figure 7**. The algorithm searches for series of consecutive upstrokes (t_{up}) and downstrokes (t_{dw}) in the capnogram. These abrupt changes are detected when the amplitude of the capnogram exceeds or goes below a fixed threshold, Th_{amp} (mmHg). Then the algorithm extracts two features, the duration between consecutive abrupt changes, considered as an estimation of expiration and inspiration intervals, D_{ex} and D_{in}. Classification of potential true ventilations is done according to a simple decision tree based on Th_{ex} and Th_{in} thresholds. If both duration features are greater than these thresholds, the ventilation is annotated at the instant when the downstroke occurs (t_{dw}).

The performance of the algorithm was evaluated in terms of its sensitivity (Se) and positive predictive value (PPV). Se was defined as the proportion of annotated ventilations that were identified by the algorithm and PPV as the proportion of detected ventilations that were true ventilations. Ventilation detection instances were matched with the gold standard annotations if they were within ±0.5 s of one another. The algorithm was first trained with a subset of 30 nondistorted episodes obtaining the maximizing Se while assuring a PPV >98%. Ventilation detection performance was reported for the remaining episodes (test set), consisting of a mixture of distorted and nondistorted episodes.

In order to assess how the ventilation rate estimation is influenced by the chest compression artifact, we computed, for each episode in the whole set, the number of ventilations given during every minute, using a 1-minute sliding window with an

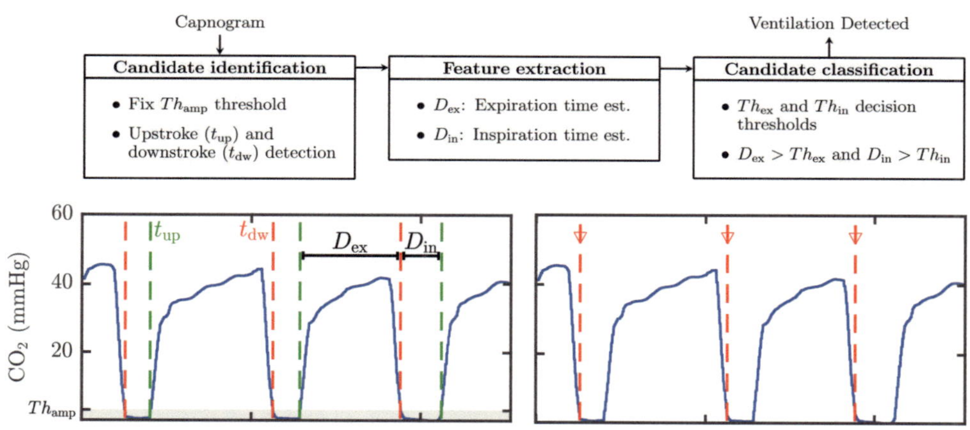

Figure 7.
The ventilation detection scheme is described in the top panel. Applying a fixed amplitude threshold Th_{amp}, the algorithm searches consecutive upstrokes (t_{up}) and downstrokes (t_{dw}) in the waveform capnography signal (bottom-left panel). Then, it extracts the duration of the intervals D_{ex} and D_{in}. Finally, features greater than the fixed duration thresholds Th_{ex} and Th_{in} are classified as true ventilations. Detected ventilations are depicted with vertical red dotted lines (bottom-right panel).

overlap factor of 1/6. Hence, ventilation rate value was updated every 10 s. Then, we compared the ventilation rate measurements estimated from the ventilation detections with those computed from the gold standard annotations. Using the computed ventilation rate per minute measurements, we also calculated the overventilation alarms obtained for a 10 min^{-1} threshold. Then, we tested the ability of our algorithm to correctly detect overventilation.

Results were reported as mean (±SD) if they passed Lilliefors normality test and as median (IQR) otherwise. Distribution of Se and PPV per record and distributions of the percent error in the estimation of ventilation rate were depicted with box plots, which graphically report median, IQR, and possible outlier values.

4.3 Characterization of chest compression artifact and ventilation detection performance

From the original dataset of 301 episodes, 23% were discarded (69 records) due to unreliable waveform capnography or TI signals. Permanent signal disconnection or saturation, capnograms without respiratory cycle variations or under 5 mmHg during the whole episode (32 records), and inability to observe ventilation fluctuations in the filtered TI signal (20 records) were some of the reasons for elimination. Remaining 232 episodes had a mean duration of 30 (±9.5) min per episode.

A total of 98 episodes (42%) were annotated as distorted. The artifact was classified into three types: type I, observed primarily during the expiratory plateau; type II, in the capnogram baseline; and type III, spanning from the plateau to the baseline. No induced chest compression oscillations were found in the slopes of phases 0 and II. **Figure 8** depicts, for each artifact type, examples of capnogram intervals observed during ongoing chest compressions. The ventilation annotation process yielded a total of 52,654 ventilation instances, with a mean of 227 (±118) ventilations per episode. Nondistorted episodes comprised 30,814 ventilations and distorted episodes 21,840 ventilations (type I, 10,119; type II, 5228; and type III, 6493).

Global Se was 96.4% and PPV was 95.0% for the whole test subset. Reported performance for nondistorted episodes was higher, Se was 99.6%, and PPV was 99.0%. However, performance decreased for the distorted subset, with values of Se and PPV of 91.9 and 89.5%, respectively. This phenomenon is highly noticeable in the case of type III episodes, where performance was drastically affected by the artifact, reporting values of Se and PPV of 77.6 and 73.5%, respectively. **Figure 9** (left panels) shows the performance results of the automated ventilation detection. **Figure 9** (right panel) shows the distribution of the unsigned percent error in the estimation of ventilation rate per episode. For the nondistorted episodes, median error was 0.9 (0–1.9)%. For the distorted subset, error was 6.3 (1.7–16.9)%. For type III episodes, error increased to 19.6 (7.7–40.3)%.

Table 1 shows the relation between the artifact type and the airway system, and the algorithm performance in the detection of overventilation alarms. Overall, type I artifact appeared in 48% of the distorted cases, type II in 21%, and type III in 31%

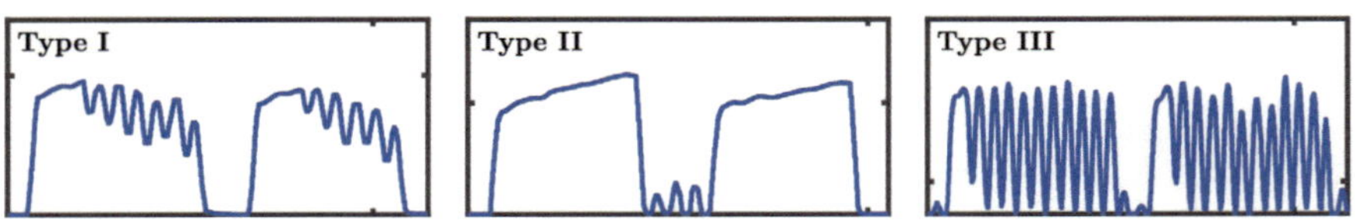

Figure 8.
Intervals of chest compression oscillations observed in OHCA capnograms during ongoing CPR: type I, located in the plateau; type II, located in the baseline; type III, spanning from the plateau to the baseline.

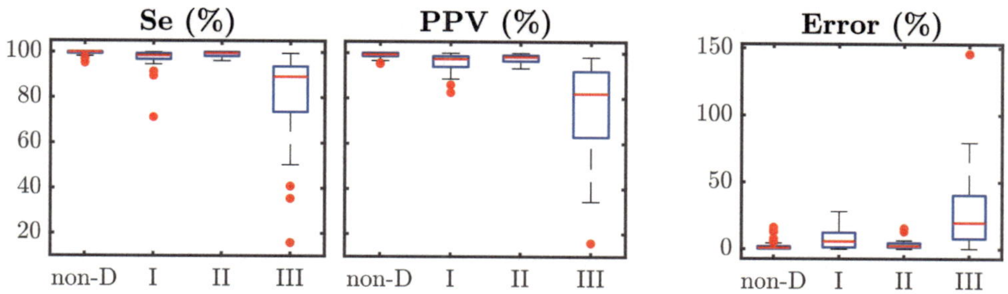

Figure 9.
Automated ventilation detection performance and error in the estimation of ventilation rate. Results are provided for all categories: non-D, nondistorted; I, type I; II, type II; and III, type III.

Group	Total	Ventilation type				Gold standard		Alarm detection	
		BVM	ETT	SGA	NA	n_{vr}	n_{ov}	Se (%)	PPV (%)
Total	232	7	149	73	3	31,760	17,901	99.1	92.6
Non-D	134	7	90	35	2	17,413	10,511	99.7	98.0
Distorted	98	0	59	38	1	14,347	7390	98.2	85.8
Type I	47	0	19	28	0	7167	3398	98.9	90.8
Type II	21	0	15	6	0	2826	1837	99.8	96.6
Type III	30	0	25	4	1	4354	2155	95.5	72.1

Non-D, nondistorted; BVM, bag valve mask; ETT, endotracheal tube; SGA, supraglottic airway; NA, not available; n_{vr}, number of ventilation rate per minute measurements annotated in the gold standard; n_{ov}, number of annotated overventilation alarms.

Table 1.
Distribution of episodes according to artifact and airway type and algorithm performance in the detection of overventilation alarms.

of them. Artifact was not present where BVM ventilation was used, although the sample was small. However, all types of artifact appeared in both advanced airways, with a higher incidence for SGA cases. In ETT cases, incidence of type III artifact was more prevalent, whereas in SGA cases, type I was more prevalent.

There was a 56.4% (17,901/31,760) of 1-minute overventilation annotated intervals. Overventilation was accurately detected in the case of nondistorted episodes, but performance decreased in the distorted group (type III), particularly with respect to PPV.

4.4 Discussion

There is a lack of evidence about the incidence and origin of the chest compression artifact. One prior study has reported the impact of these induced oscillations on the capnogram during OHCA CPR. In this work, published as a conference abstract, Idris et al. [33] reported the appearance of oscillations in 154 episodes from a total of 210 OHCA records (73.3%). In our study, with a similar number of OHCA episodes (232 vs. 210), we found a lower incidence of distorted capnograms (42%). This could be explained by a different criterion for distorted episode classification.

Ventilation rate guidance is one of the emphasized advantages of capnography during OCHA episodes. However, the presence of fast oscillations in the capnogram during ongoing CPR may limit rescuers since distorted capnograms are difficult to interpret. Performed analyses demonstrated the negative impact of this artifact in the detection of ventilations. Se and PPV were above 95%, and ventilation rate estimation errors were minimal for all the nondistorted episodes, but detection performance significantly decreased in the presence of oscillations. Thus, a reliable ventilation guidance would not be feasible for those OHCA patients.

Overventilation was common in our database: 56.4% of the annotated ventilation rates were above the recommended 10 breaths per minute. Sensitivity for alarm detection was high for all episodes (nondistorted and distorted). However, the algorithm showed a tendency to overestimate ventilation rate in the presence of chest compression oscillations, where PPV values were low. Induced oscillations spanning from the plateau to the baseline impeded a reliable detection of true ventilation CO_2 concentration changes. Hence, the presence of artifact in the waveform capnography caused many false ventilation detections.

5. Suppression of chest compression artifact during CPR

In Section 2 we quantitatively confirmed the nature of the oscillations, with a single frequency matching the chest compression rate, suggesting that the artifact is directly caused by ongoing chest compressions during CPR. In this context, we hypothesized that automatic ventilation detection would improve if the oscillations induced by chest compressions could be successfully removed from the capnogram. Our next step was designing chest compression artifact suppression techniques, exploring different alternatives.

5.1 Frequency domain filtering techniques

The following section describes the filtering techniques used for the suppression of the chest compression oscillations induced in the capnogram. We studied three different alternatives: a simple fixed-coefficient filter and two computationally intensive adaptive filtering techniques. To assess the goodness of the filter, we computed the performance using an automated capnogram-based ventilation detector after filtering OHCA capnograms. We also evaluated the improvement in ventilation rate measurement and in overventilation alarm detection. Then, we compared these results with those obtained before filtering, described previously in Section 4.4.

5.1.1 Fixed-coefficient filter

The spectral analysis performed on OHCA capnograms (see Section 3, **Figure 5**) suggests that a sensible strategy to suppress the oscillations induced by chest compressions in the capnogram would be to use a simple fixed-coefficient filter that suppresses the spectral content of the capnogram above 1 Hz (compression rate above 60 cpm). To that end, after analyzing the spectral characteristics of several waveform capnography and CD signals, we developed a digital infinite impulse response low-pass Butterworth filter (8th order, cutoff frequency of 1.5 Hz).

5.1.2 Adaptive filtering

Efficacy of the fixed-coefficient filter may be affected by the variability of chest compression and ventilation rates during CPR [17, 18, 30, 42]. In the literature, filters adjusted in time, according to the varying characteristics of the artifact, have been extensively used to suppress oscillations in the electrocardiogram induced by chest compressions [43–46]. In this study, we designed two adaptive filtering configurations, an open-loop and a closed-loop adaptive filter [47]. Both techniques used the annotated chest compression instances, obtained from the CD signal as a reference to adjust the parameters of the adaptive filters. To do so, chest compression instances were annotated at the local minima as shown in **Figure 6** (top panel), corresponding to the maximum depth achieved for each chest compression. For more details of the adaptive filters, see Ref. [48].

Open-loop adaptive filter. This technique is based on the adaptive adjustment of a stop-band Butterworth filter whose central frequency is adaptively adjusted to the chest compression rate. Average chest compression rate was estimated in 2-s nonoverlapped windows, using the annotated chest compression instances. Thus, filter parameters were updated every 2 s.

Closed-loop adaptive filter. In our approach, the required reference signal was modeled as a pure cosine wave of time-varying amplitude and phase, estimating the instantaneous chest compression rate from the chest compression instances. In this configuration, the artifact is adaptively estimated and subtracted from the capnogram, resulting in an equivalent notch filter capable of adaptively tracking the chest compression oscillation frequency.

5.1.3 Results

The three proposed filter schemes performed similarly, reporting favorable global Se and PPV values well above 97 and 96%, respectively, for the distorted episodes, and maintaining the performance for nondistorted episodes. For this reason, and trying to keep this section as simple as possible, results for the closed-loop filter are reported. These results are representative of the three approaches. Readers are encouraged to see full results in Ref. [48].

Globally, Se/PPV improved from 96.4/95.0% before filtering to 98.2/98.3%. Performance improvement for type III episodes was remarkably higher, with Se/PPV improving from a low 77.6/73.5% to 95.5/95.5%. **Figure 10** (left panels) shows, for each artifact type, the distribution of Se and PPV per episode, before and after filtering. In the case of type III episodes, the high dispersion in performance was drastically reduced after artifact suppression. Box plots in **Figure 10** (right panel) show the distribution of error in the estimation of ventilation rate before and after filtering. In the same way, estimation error for type III episodes noticeably decreased after filtering.

Table 2 shows the performance improvement in the detection of overventilation. Globally, Se/PPV improved from 99.1/92.6% before filtering to 97.9/98.0%

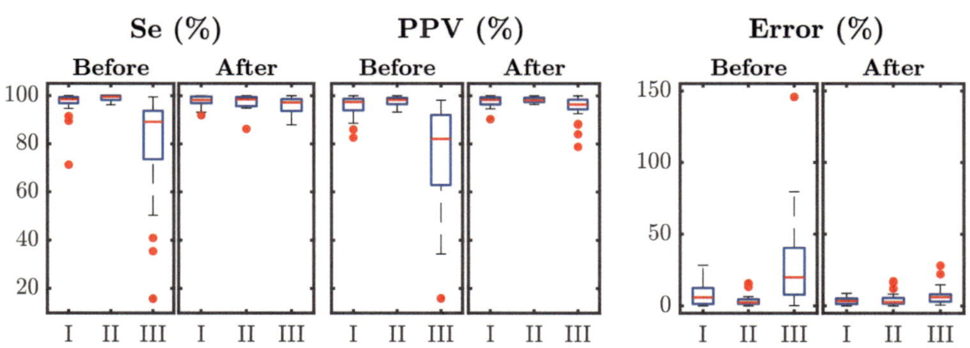

Figure 10.
Se and PPV distribution per episode before and after filtering (left). Distribution of the unsigned error in the ventilation rate estimation (right). Results are provided for each artifact category: I, type I artifact; II, type II artifact; and III, type III artifact.

Group	Gold standard		Before		After	
	n_{vr}	n_{ov}	Se (%)	PPV (%)	Se (%)	PPV (%)
Total	31,760	17,901	99.1	92.6	97.9	98.0
Nondistorted	17,413	10,511	99.7	98.0	98.9	98.9
Distorted	14,347	7390	98.2	85.8	96.3	96.6
Type I	7167	3398	98.9	90.8	98.0	97.0
Type II	2826	1837	99.8	96.6	95.2	98.3
Type III	4354	2155	95.5	72.1	94.8	94.2

n_{vr}, number of ventilation rate per minute measurements annotated in the gold standard; n_{ov}, number of annotated overventilation alarms.

Table 2.
Performance in the detection of overventilation alarms before and after filtering.

after filtering. Although the improvement for the distorted group was noticeable in all cases, improvement was remarkably higher for type III episodes, with Se/PPV of 95.5/72.1% before and 94.8/94.2% after filtering.

A graphical example of the closed-loop filtering approach is illustrated in **Figure 11**. The raw capnogram is depicted by the solid gray line and the resulting waveform capnography after filtering by the solid blue superimposed to the raw capnogram. Each vertical dashed red line indicates a detection of ventilation given by the automated ventilation detector.

5.1.4 Discussion

The presented filtering techniques were designed to preprocess the raw capnogram before applying the ventilation detection algorithm with the aim of improving automated ventilation detection. Although the closed-loop approach showed a great balance in Se and PPV improvement, none of the techniques showed a distinctive superiority in terms of performance. Since chest compression rates tend to vary during CPR, one could expect that adaptive filters would present better results than a simple fixed-coefficient filter, but this was not the case. This could be explained in part because chest compression rate is usually ten times greater than ventilation rate; thus spectral information is far away from one another. The selection of the filtering strategy could be analyzed in terms of simplicity and computational burden. Consequently, applying a simple fixed-coefficient filter to remove the chest compression artifact seems to be adequate.

As illustrated in **Figure 11**, resulting waveform capnography obtained after filtering approximates the mean peak-to-peak amplitude of the artifact. After

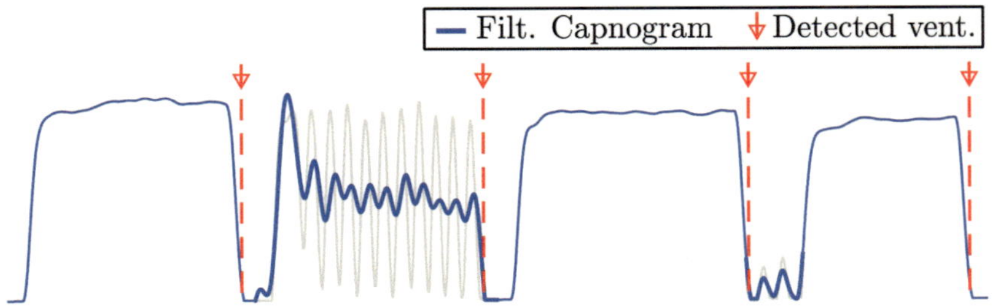

Figure 11.
Example of filtering performance. Original capnogram with clean and distorted respiration cycles is depicted by the solid gray line. Filtered capnogram (in blue) superimposed to the original capnogram. Detected ventilations are depicted with vertical dashed red lines.

filtering, output capnogram waveform hinders the $ETCO_2$ measurement and a reliable analysis of $ETCO_2$ trends. Thus, clinicians may still find the capnogram difficult to interpret. Removing the artifact to improve ventilation detection and at the same time preserving the capnogram tracing, which favors clinical interpretation, require the development of new suppressing techniques.

5.2 Time-domain artifact suppression technique

In the previous section, we proposed a solution to suppress chest compression artifact from the waveform capnography using different filtering approaches. Although the automated detection of ventilations was improved, filtered capnograms were far from being clinically reliable.

This section explores an alternative method to remove chest compression oscillations from the waveform capnography signal. This technique was designed to improve ventilation detection focusing on the real tracing preservation. Again, performance metrics previously described in the chapter were used for quantitatively assessing the goodness of the method. This study was conducted using the test subset described in Section 4.4.

5.2.1 Envelope detection algorithm

The principle of this artifact suppression technique relies on the hypothesis that the envelope of the waveform capnography signal could be a clinically reliable estimation of the CO_2 concentration tracing produced by ventilations. Due to artifact morphology and location variability reported in Section 4, the algorithm determines how to extract the envelope of the waveform capnography dividing its operation into low and high CO_2 concentration intervals.

A graphical explanation of the method's performance is given in **Figure 12**. To extract the upper envelope of the capnogram (dashed blue line), the algorithm detects the local maxima values (downward arrowheads) during the plateau phase and applies a smoothing filter. Then, in order to extract the lower envelope (dotted blue line), local minima values (upward arrowheads) are detected during the capnogram baseline. A detailed explanation of the algorithm is provided in Ref. [49].

5.2.2 Results

Globally, performance of the automated ventilation detection in terms of Se/PPV improved from 96.4/95.0% to 98.5/98.3% after artifact suppression.

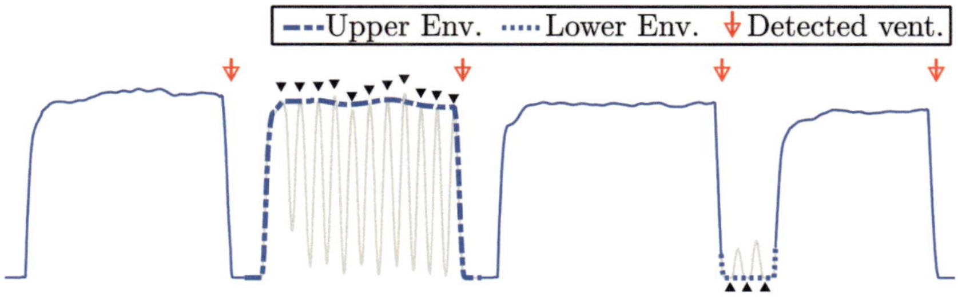

Figure 12.
Chest compression artifact suppression example. A distorted capnogram interval is depicted by the gray line. The blue line illustrates the waveform capnography envelope extraction process. Upper envelope (dashed blue line) is extracted through the detection of each local maxima (downward arrowheads), and lower envelope (dotted blue line) is extracted through the detection of each local minima (upward arrowheads). Detected ventilations are depicted with vertical red arrows.

Performance for nondistorted episodes stayed stable, whereas Se/PPV for distorted episodes increased noticeably, from 91.9/89.5% to 98.0/97.3%. As it happens with previous filtering methods, performance improved more in type III episodes, with Se/PPV increasing from 77.6/73.5% to 97.1/96.1%. **Figure 13** (left panels) depicts trough box plots, for each artifact type, the distribution of Se and PPV per episode given by the automated ventilation detector. In general, median values of both performance metrics increased after artifact suppression, and dispersion was reduced for all groups. These improvements were more noticeable for type III episodes. Performance regarding ventilation rate estimation is shown in **Figure 13** (right panel), in which box plots depict the distribution of the error before and after applying the suppression method. Errors were reduced in all groups, but again, improvements in case of type III episodes were noticeably higher.

Results after artifact suppression in the detection of excessive ventilation rates are reported in **Table 3**. In this case, Se stayed almost stable with a higher increase for PPV values. For the distorted subset, Se/PPV was 98.8/86.7% before and 98.4/96.3% after suppressing the artifact, implying a reduction in false overventilation alarms. Once again, most remarkable results were obtained for type III episodes, with a slight increase in Se, but with PPV increasing from 73.9 to 93.6% after artifact suppression.

Finally, performance of the suppression method is illustrated in **Figure 14**. The raw capnogram is depicted by a solid gray line and the resulting waveform capnography by a solid blue line superimposed to the raw capnogram.

5.2.3 Discussion

Filtering methods to remove the oscillations from the capnogram, described in Section 4, improved ventilation detection accuracy. However, filtered capnograms do not accurately represent the CO_2 concentration in intervals where the artifact appeared. In this section, a method that tries to preserve the waveform capnography has been proposed. Automated detection of ventilation instances, as well as estimation of ventilation rate and detection of overventilation, improved after artifact suppression. Results obtained with this method were similar or even better than the result reported for several filtering methods (Section 4).

The idea of "preserving the capnogram waveform" refers to the extraction of a clinically useful capnogram. We visually analyzed several capnogram segments in our database showing consecutive intervals with nondistorted and distorted ventilations (**Figure 14**). In most cases, the envelope of the distorted capnogram

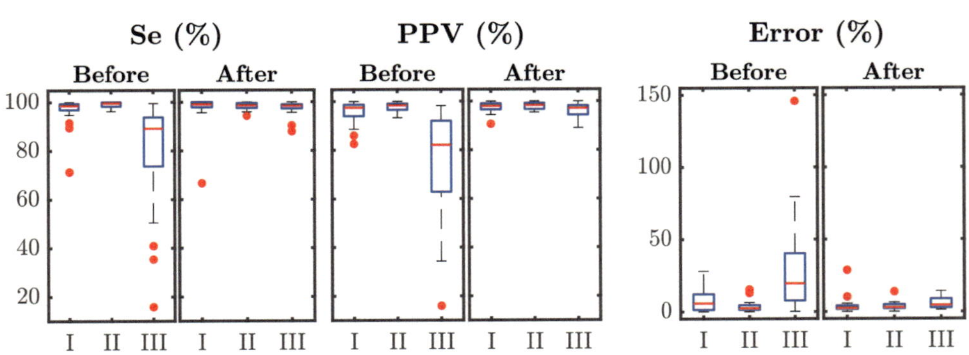

Figure 13.
Se and PPV distribution per episode before and after artifact suppression method (left). Distribution of the unsigned error in the ventilation rate estimation (right). Results are provided for each artifact category: I, type I artifact; II, type II artifact; and III, type III artifact.

Group	Total	Gold standard		Before		After	
		n_{vr}	n_{ov}	Se (%)	PPV (%)	Se (%)	PPV (%)
Total	202	25,833	15,237	99.3	93.1	98.9	97.8
Nondistorted	119	14,889	8873	99.7	98.2	99.3	98.9
Distorted	83	10,944	6364	98.8	86.7	98.4	96.3
Type I	42	5823	2961	99.1	90.7	98.7	97.2
Type II	16	2160	1570	99.8	97.8	97.5	97.7
Type III	25	2961	1833	97.2	73.9	98.7	93.6

n_{vr}, number of ventilation rate per minute measurements annotated in the gold standard; n_{ov}, number of annotated overventilation alarms.

Table 3.
Overventilation alarm detection performance before and after applying the artifact suppression method.

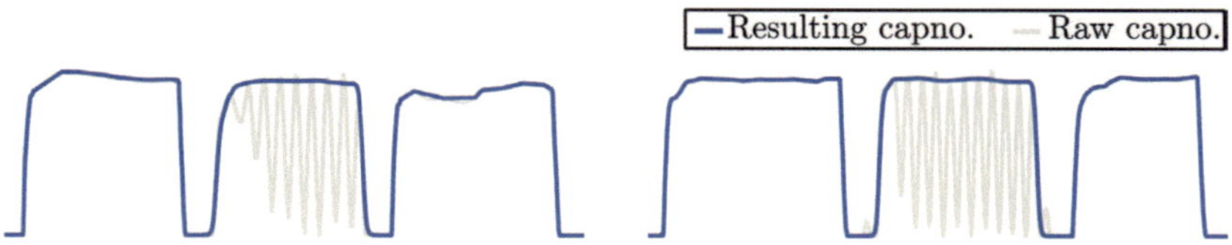

Figure 14.
Examples of artifact suppression method performance. Original capnogram with clean and distorted respiration cycles is depicted by the solid gray line. Filtered capnogram (in blue) superimposed to the original capnogram.

resembled the CO_2 tracing observed in the preceding and following undistorted respiratory cycles. Therefore, this method could enhance capnographs not accounting for the chest compression artifact effect.

6. Conclusions

Current resuscitation guidelines emphasize the use of waveform capnography during CPR in order to enhance CPR quality and improve patient outcomes. However, the first study presented in this chapter showed that ventilation rate and overventilation prevention were compromised by the high incidence of chest compression artifact. The appearance of artifact during ongoing CPR is unpredictable, and thus suppression algorithms that continuously process the raw capnogram could be a great approach for waveform capnography enhancement. All artifact suppression approaches yielded good performance in terms of sensitivity and positive predictive value figures of merit. However, the time-domain alternative was the only one that enhanced the capnogram tracing, favoring its interpretation during CPR. The implementation of artifact suppression techniques in current capnographs could increase the use of capnography in OHCA episodes, which could in turn contribute to improving CPR quality.

Acknowledgements

This work received financial support from the Basque Government (Basque Country, Spain) through the project IT1087-16 and the predoctoral research grant PRE-2017-2-0201.

The authors thank the TVF&R emergency medical service providers for collecting the out-of-hospital cardiac arrest episodes used in this study.

Conflict of interest

The authors declare no conflicts of interest.

Author details

Mikel Leturiondo*, Sofía Ruiz de Gauna, José Julio Gutiérrez, Digna M. González-Otero, Jesus M. Ruiz, Luis A. Leturiondo and Purificación Saiz
University of the Basque Country (UPV/EHU), Bilbao, Spain

*Address all correspondence to: mikel.leturiondo@ehu.eus

References

[1] Mehra R. Global public health problem of sudden cardiac death. Journal of Electrocardiology. 2007;**40**(6):S118-S122

[2] Katritsis DG, Gersh BJ, Camm AJ. A clinical perspective on sudden cardiac death. Arrhythmia & Electrophysiology Review. 2016;**5**(3):177

[3] Myerburg RJ, Kessler KM, Castellanos A. Sudden cardiac death. Structure, function, and time-dependence of risk. Circulation. 1992;**85**(1 Suppl):I2-I10

[4] Kannel WB, Schatzkin A. Sudden death: Lessons from subsets in population studies. Journal of the American College of Cardiology. 1985;**5**(6 Supplement 1):141B-149B

[5] Atwood C, Eisenberg MS, Herlitz J, Rea TD. Incidence of EMS-treated out-of-hospital cardiac arrest in Europe. Resuscitation. 2005;**67**(1):75-80

[6] Nichol G, Baker D. The epidemiology of sudden death. In: Paradir NA, Halperin HR, Kern KB, Wenzel V, Chamberlain D, editors. Cardiac Arrest: Science and Practice of Resuscitation Medicine. Cambridge: Cambridge University Press; 2007. pp. 26-50

[7] Soar J, Nolan JP, Böttiger BW, Perkins GD, Lott C, Carli P, et al. European Resuscitation Council guidelines for resuscitation 2015. Section 3. Adult advanced life support. Resuscitation. 2015;**95**:100-147

[8] Link MS, Berkow LC, Kudenchuk PJ, Halperin HR, Hess EP, Moitra VK, et al. 2015 American Heart Association Guidelines Update for Cardiopulmonary Resuscitation and Emergency Cardiovascular Care. Part 7: Adult advanced cardiovascular life support. Circulation. 2015;**132** (18 suppl 2):S444-S464

[9] Idris AH, Guffey D, Aufderheide TP, Brown S, Morrison LJ, Nichols P, et al. Relationship between chest compression rates and outcomes from cardiac arrest. Circulation. 2012;**125**:3004-3012

[10] Edelson DP, Abella BS, Kramer-Johansen J, Wik L, Myklebust H, Barry AM, et al. Effects of compression depth and pre-shock pauses predict defibrillation failure during cardiac arrest. Resuscitation. 2006;**71**(2):137-145

[11] Kramer-Johansen J, Myklebust H, Wik L, Fellows B, Svensson L, Sørebø H, et al. Quality of out-of-hospital cardiopulmonary resuscitation with real time automated feedback: A prospective interventional study. Resuscitation. 2006;**71**(3):283-292

[12] Monsieurs KG, Nolan JP, Bossaert LL, Greif R, Maconochie IK, Nikolaou NI, et al. European resuscitation council guidelines for resuscitation 2015: Section 1. Executive summary. Resuscitation. 2015;**95**:1-80

[13] Berg RA, Hemphill R, Abella BS, Aufderheide TP, Cave DM, Hazinski MF, et al. Part 5: Adult basic life support: 2010 American Heart Association Guidelines for Cardiopulmonary Resuscitation and Emergency Cardiovascular Care. Circulation. 2010;**122**(18 Suppl 3):S685-S705

[14] Pitts S, Kellermann AL. Hyperventilation during cardiac arrest. Lancet. 2004;**364**(9431):313-315

[15] Benoit JL, Prince DK, Wang HE. Mechanisms linking advanced airway management and cardiac arrest outcomes. Resuscitation. 2015;**93**:124-127

[16] Aufderheide TP, Sigurdsson G, Pirrallo RG, Yannopoulos D, McKnite S, von Briesen C, et al.

Hyperventilation-induced hypotension during cardiopulmonary resuscitation. Circulation. 2004;**109**(16):1960-1965

[17] O'Neill JF, Deakin CD. Do we hyperventilate cardiac arrest patients? Resuscitation. 2007;**73**(1):82-85

[18] Maertens VL, De Smedt LE, Lemoyne S, Huybrechts SA, Wouters K, Kalmar AF, et al. Patients with cardiac arrest are ventilated two times faster than guidelines recommend: an observational prehospital study using tracheal pressure measurement. Resuscitation. 2013;**84**(7):921-926

[19] Yannopoulos D, McKnite S, Aufderheide TP, Sigurdsson G, Pirrallo RG, Benditt D, et al. Effects of incomplete chest wall decompression during cardiopulmonary resuscitation on coronary and cerebral perfusion pressures in a porcine model of cardiac arrest. Resuscitation. 2005;**64**(3):363-372

[20] Aufderheide TP, Lurie KG. Death by hyperventilation: A common and life-threatening problem during cardiopulmonary resuscitation. Critical Care Medicine. 2004;**32**(9):S345-S351

[21] Silvestri S, Ralls GA, Krauss B, Thundiyil J, Rothrock SG, Senn A, et al. The effectiveness of out-of-hospital use of continuous end-tidal carbon dioxide monitoring on the rate of unrecognized misplaced intubation within a regional emergency medical services system. Annals of Emergency Medicine. 2005;**45**(5):497-503

[22] Qvigstad E, Kramer-Johansen J, Tømte Ø, Skålhegg T, Sørensen Ø, Sunde K, et al. Clinical pilot study of different hand positions during manual chest compressions monitored with capnography. Resuscitation. 2013;**84**(9):1203-1207

[23] Pokorná M, Nečas E, Kratochvíl J, Skřipský R, Andrlík M, Franěk O. A sudden increase in partial pressure end-tidal carbon dioxide (PETCO2) at the moment of return of spontaneous circulation. The Journal of Emergency Medicine. 2010;**38**(5):614-621

[24] Kodali BS, Urman RD, et al. Capnography during cardiopulmonary resuscitation: Current evidence and future directions. Journal of Emergencies, Trauma, and Shock. 2014;**7**(4):332

[25] Touma O, Davies M. The prognostic value of end tidal carbon dioxide during cardiac arrest: A systematic review. Resuscitation. 2013;**84**(11):1470-1479

[26] Jaffe MB. Infrared measurement of carbon dioxide in the human breath: "Breathe-through" devices from Tyndall to the present day. Anesthesia and Analgesia. 2008;**107**(3):890-904

[27] Bhavani-Shankar K, Philip JH. Defining segments and phases of a time capnogram. Anesthesia and Analgesia. 2000;**91**(4):973-977

[28] Gravenstein JS, Jaffe MB, Gravenstein N, Paulus DA. Capnography. In: Gravenstein JS, editor. Clinical Perspectives. Cambridge: Cambridge University Press; 2011. pp. 6-9

[29] Pantazopoulos C, Xanthos T, Pantazopoulos I, Papalois A, Kouskouni E, Iacovidou N. A review of carbon dioxide monitoring during adult cardiopulmonary resuscitation. Heart, Lung & Circulation. 2015;**24**(11):1053-1061

[30] Meaney PA, Bobrow BJ, Mancini ME, et al. Cardiopulmonary resuscitation quality: Improving cardiac resuscitation outcomes both inside and outside the hospital: A consensus statement from the American Heart Association. Circulation. 2013;**128**(4):417-435

[31] Takla G, Petre JH, Doyle DJ, Horibe M, Gopakumaran B. The problem of artifactsin patient monitor data during surgery: A clinical and methodological review. Anesthesia and Analgesia. 2006;**103**(5):1196-1204

[32] Herry CL, Townsend D, Green GC, Bravi A, Seely AJE. Segmentation and classi-fication of capnograms: Application in respiratory variability analysis. Physiological Measurement. 2014;**35**(12):2343

[33] Idris AH, Daya M, Owens P, et al. High incidence of chest compression oscillations associated with capnography during out-of-hospital cardiopulmonary resuscitation. Circulation. 2010;**122**:A83

[34] Deakin CD, O'Neill JF, Tabor T. Does compression-only cardiopulmonary resuscitation generate adequate passive ventilation during cardiac arrest? Resuscitation. 2007;**75**(1):53-59

[35] Vanwulpen M, Wolfskeil M, Duchatelet C, Monsieurs K, Idrissi SH. Quantifying inspiratory volumes generated by manual chest compressions during resuscitation in the prehospital setting. Resuscitation. 2017;**118**:e18

[36] Idris AH, Banner MJ, Wenzel V, Fuerst RS, Becker LB, Melker RJ. Ventilation caused by external chest compression is unable to sustain effective gas exchange during CPR: A comparison with mechanical ventilation. Resuscitation. 1994;**28**(2):143-150

[37] Leturiondo M, de Gauna SR, Ruiz JM, Gutiérrez JJ, Leturiondo LA, González-Otero DM, et al. Influence of chest compression artefact on capnogram-based ventilation detection during out-of-hospital cardiopulmonary resuscitation. Resuscitation. 2018;**124**:63-68

[38] Raimondi M, Savastano S, Pamploni G, Molinari S, Degani A, Belliato M. End-tidal carbon dioxide monitoring and load band device for mechanical cardio-pulmonary resuscitation: Never trust the numbers, believe at the curves. Resuscitation. 2016;**103**:e9-e10

[39] Pellis T, Bisera J, Tang W, Weil MH. Expanding automatic external defibrillators to include automated detection of cardiac, respiratory, and cardiorespiratory arrest. Critical Care Medicine. 2002;**30**(4):S176-S178

[40] Losert H, Risdal M, Sterz F, Nysaether J, KoÈhler K, Eftestøl T, et al. Thoracic impedance changes measured via defibrillator pads can monitor ventilation in critically ill patients and during cardiopulmonary resuscitation. Critical Care Medicine. 2006;**34**(9):2399-2405

[41] Edelson DP, Eilevstjønn J, Weidman EK, Retzer E, Hoek TLV, Abella BS. Capnography and chest-wall impedance algorithms for ventilation detection during cardiopulmonary resuscitation. Resuscitation. 2010;**81**(3):317-322

[42] Abella BS, Sandbo N, Vassilatos P, Alvarado JP, O'hearn N, Wigder HN, et al. Chest compression rates during cardiopulmonary resuscitation are suboptimal: A prospective study during in-hospital cardiac arrest. Circulation. 2005;**111**(4):428-434

[43] Aase SO, Eftestøl T, Husøy JH, Sunde K, Steen PA. CPR artifact removal from human ECG using optimal multichannel filtering. IEEE Transactions on Biomedical Engineering. 2000;**47**(11):1440-1449

[44] Eilevstjønn J, Eftestøl T, Aase SO, Myklebust H, Husøy JH, Steen PA. Feasibility of shock advice analysis during CPR through removal of CPR artefacts from the human ECG. Resuscitation. 2004;**61**(2):131-141

[45] Gong Y, Chen B, Li Y. A review of the performance of artifact filtering algorithms for cardiopulmonary resuscitation. Journal of Healthcare Engineering. 2013;**4**(2):185-202

[46] Ruiz de Gauna S, Irusta U, Ruiz J, Ayala U, Aramendi E, Eftestøl T. Rhythm analysis during cardiopulmonary resuscitation: Past, present, and future. BioMed Research International. 2014;**2014**:1-13

[47] Widrow B, Stearns SD. Adaptive Signal Processing. Vol. 1. Englewood Cliffs, NJ: Prentice-Hall, Inc; 1985. p. 491

[48] Gutiérrez JJ, Leturiondo M, Ruiz de Gauna S, Ruiz JM, Leturiondo LA, et al. Enhancing ventilation detection during cardiopulmonary resuscitation by filtering chest compression artifact from the capnography waveform. PLoS One. 2018;**13**(8):e0201565

[49] Ruiz de Gauna S, Leturiondo M, Gutiérrez JJ, Ruiz JM, González-Otero DM, Russell JK, et al. Enhancement of capnogram waveform in the presence of chest compression artefact during cardiopulmonary resuscitation. Resuscitation. 2018;**133**:53-58

Chapter 4

Characteristics of Acute Myocardial Damage in Uzbekistan: Data Register "RACSMI-Uz"

Nagaeva Gulnora

Abstract

In 2015, a register of acute coronary events (acute coronary syndrome and acute myocardial infarction) was carried out in one of the districts of the city of Tashkent. The study included 782 patients, of which 491 (63.7%) were analyzed (hereinafter 100%) and the remaining 291 (36.3%) were dead (according to the civil registry office). The average age of patients was 58.3 ± 7.9 years. The features of the patient's nosological structures were established separately for men and women when admitted to hospital and discharged from hospital, which will make it possible to further adjust the tactics of management of these categories of patients, taking into account their gender and other uncompensated risk factors.

Keywords: acute coronary syndrome, acute myocardial infarction, register, risk factors, men, women, arterial hypertension, obesity, diabetes

1. Introduction

The emergence of epidemiology as a science made it possible to formulate the basic principles of conducting research, which make it possible to obtain real information about the prevalence of diseases, the characteristics of their occurrence and course, outcomes, etc. [1]. One of the first major epidemiological studies in the field of cardiology was the well-known Framingham study, which revealed the main factors contributing to the development of cardiovascular diseases (CVD), as well as the role of these diseases in mortality rates [2, 3].

At the same time, epidemiological studies are not the most successful way to study a particular disease, especially when it comes to studying the characteristics of its course, outcomes, the treatment used, and its effectiveness. In the mid-twentieth century, it became clear that the most accurate method for obtaining information about the real clinical course of the disease, its outcomes, etc. in certain regions or even in individual medical institutions is the so-called registers, which are an organized system for collecting information about patients having a specific disease or receiving a specific treatment [1, 4].

For several decades, the registers of acute myocardial infarction (AMI) and, more recently, the registers of acute coronary syndrome (ACS) are regularly held in different countries of the world, and their scale varies from individual clinics (and even departments in clinics) to large regions, whole countries, and even groups of countries (international registries). Perhaps the most famous are registers such as Global Registry of Acute Coronary Events Project (GRACE), registers of the European Society of Cardiology (EHS-ACS-I, EHS-ACS-II), and CRUSADE register [5]. However, these registries do not allow a comprehensive assessment of the quality of diagnosis and treatment of arterial hypertension (AH), coronary heart disease (CHD), chronic heart failure, diabetes mellitus (DM), their combinations, etc. in actual clinical practice, to determine the structure of risk factors (RFs) and comorbidities in this category of patients.

Individual attention is required for patients with concomitant disorders of carbohydrate metabolism, in particular with the presence of DM. According to the International Diabetes Federation (IDF, 2014), at present, diabetes affects 400 million people in the world, and by 2035, their number will increase to 600 million people. It is known that DM increases the risk of developing CVD by a factor of 2–4, and mortality with a combination of CVD and DM increases four to five times [6, 7]. The paradox of DM is the increase in CVD in women and the lack of reduction in the growth of these diseases in men, in countries that have achieved significant success in the treatment of coronary artery disease (CHD) [8]. The combination of a whole cluster of rapid development and progression of atherosclerosis based on insulin resistance—hyperglycemia, dyslipidemia, AH—allowed the expert committee of the US National Cholesterol Education Program (NCEP) to equate type 2 diabetes to CHD. Today, DM is considered as equivalent to the presence of clinically significant CVD [9]. Nevertheless, against the background of modern technologies and rapidly developing interventional treatment methods for acute forms of CHD, the attention of clinicians is more focused on the treatment of the disease itself than on the causes of it or RF of its development. Used in modern clinical practice, standards for the treatment of CHD (β-blockers, BAB; angiotensin-converting enzyme inhibitors, inhibitors ACE inhibitors; aspirin, statins, antiplatelet agents, etc.), according to numerous randomized clinical trials [10], have proven to be effective, safe, and positive prognosis in this category of patients. However, there remains the question of how these drugs are regularly and consistently used by the patients themselves and what impact this has on the further course of the disease and the condition of the patients. From this perspective, the real evaluation of therapy received by patients in such practical health conditions is of great scientific and practical interest.

The foregoing implies the relevance and practical significance of the creation of the register for acute coronary syndrome and acute myocardial infarction in Uzbekistan (RACSMI-Uz), with the inclusion of patients with similar diagnoses, as well as an assessment of the interdependence of these RFs and gender characteristics. On the territory of Uzbekistan, such registers were not previously conducted; therefore, this study is not only practically interesting and relevant but also in demand.

2. Own results of research

2.1 Material and methods of research

The research material was created and processed, in accordance with the developed register protocol (map-register), a database of personal data of patients hospitalized with a diagnosis of ACS/AMI for 1 calendar (2015) year.

Data analysis of all patients with ACS/AMI during the register implied that the following conditions were:

- Patients must meet inclusion criteria.
- Patient involvement should not affect the approaches to his treatment.
- The inclusion of the patient in the register must be accompanied by his registration in the database with filling in the "register card" for each patient.

2.1.1 Inclusion criteria

The register included patients aged from 18 to 70 years old who applied to the emergency medical service, hospitalized in relevant hospitals for ACS/AMI.

- ACS and AMI were diagnosed based on generally accepted criteria.

2.1.1.1 Clinical characteristic

Complaints of patients with acute coronary insufficiency include the following:

- Frequent heartbeat.
- The pain, which is usually described as pressure, squeezing or burning in the entire left half of the chest and can be transmitted to the neck, shoulder, jaw, rear upper region of the body and to the left arm.
- Dyspnea on exertion.
- Diaphoresis (excessive sweating), due to the irritant effect of the sympathetic trunk.
- Nausea, due to stimulation of the vagus nerve.
- Severe fatigue, even with minimal exertion.

2.1.1.2 ECG diagnosis

WHO experts have suggested distinguishing between certain ECG changes, indicating a myocardial infarction, and ambiguous ECG changes that allow to suspect myocardial infarction [11]. The following ECG changes are diagnostically significant:

- New or repeated lifting of the ST segment by 1 mm or more in at least two adjacent chest leads or by 2 mm or more in two leads from the extremities. Depression of the ST segment in leads V1–V3 is considered as the equivalent of ST-elevation with suspected IM posterior localization.
- The emergence of new or deepening of existing pathological teeth Q (duration ≥30 ms and depth ≥ 1 mm in two adjacent chest leads or in two leads from the extremities). An increase in the amplitude of the R-wave in leads V1–V3 is considered as the equivalent of the Q wave in cases of suspected IM of posterior location.
- Acute blockade of the left bundle of His.
- Interpretation of the ECG dynamics against the background of changes caused by previous MI, especially in its acute period, can be very difficult. Therefore,

crucial in the diagnosis of recurrent MI acquire serum markers of necrosis. Among them, the leading role belongs to CPK, CPK-MB, and myoglobin but not troponins, since elevated levels of the latter in the blood persist for a long time and may mask their possible new rises. Re-elevation of CPK-MB above normal or 50% higher than the previous peak, or repeated elevation of total CPK or myoglobin twice as high as the upper limit of normal, allows a sufficient degree of confidence to diagnose a relapse of a heart attack.

2.1.1.3 Dynamics of myocardial damage markers

In our study, we evaluated troponin-T in a qualitative manner using a special indicator. Troponin-T is a myocardic protein, and its elevated blood level is diagnosed 2–3 h after a heart attack. The maximum amount of protein is detected 10 h after the onset of the attack. Troponin-T is preserved in the blood during a heart attack at a very high level for quite a long time—up to 7 days. Troponin-T refers to cardiospecific markers, which make it possible to determine undiagnosed infarction that has passed in a patient without clearly expressed symptoms and who does not have pronounced signs according to the ECG results. The test is very simple to use. Two to three drops of the patient's blood are applied to a special indicator. You can evaluate the result of the study in 10–15 min. When staining two bands on the indicator, we can conclude that the patient suffered a heart attack. If only one lane turned out to be colored, then health problems are caused by other causes and pathologies [12].

2.1.2 Exclusion criteria

- Age under 18 and over 70 years

2.1.2.1 Statistical analysis

Statistical processing of the results was carried out on a Pentium-IV personal computer using the STATISTICA 6 software package. Calculate the arithmetic mean (M) and root-mean-square (standard) deviation (SD).

In our study to avoid statistical inaccuracy, the analysis was accompanied by a check on the normal distribution of clinical signs.

To compare the arithmetic means of the two groups, the t-student test was used. To assess the presence of relationships between indicators, a correlation analysis was performed with the calculation of the Pearson correlation coefficient. To analyze the reliability of differences between qualitative signs, the $\chi 2$ criterion was used.

2.1.2.2 Ethical aspects

The study was conducted in accordance with the principles of the Helsinki Declaration.

2.2 Comparative analysis of the results of the register "RACSMI-Uz" depending on gender

For a comparative analysis of clinical and anamnestic data, as well as determining patient adherence to medical recommendations, depending on gender two groups of patients were allocated: 1g = 243 male patients and 2g = 206 female patients.

The study found that men with ACS/AMI were younger than women. The age difference was due to the fact that among men, patients younger than 50 years prevailed. Namely, the age category up to 40 years in the group of men was 3.3% and in the group of women = 0.5% (p = 0.076 и $\chi2$ = 2157); the number of men aged 41–50 years was 20.6% and among women = 12.1% (p = 0.024 и $\chi2$ = 5116).

On the contrary, age categories 51–60 years and 61+ were priority for females. In particular, the number of men aged 51–60 turned out to be 36.2%, and the number of women = 40.3%; the number of men in the 60+ category turned out to be 39.9% and for women = 47.1%. This was confirmed during the correlation analysis (**Figure 1**).

The calculation of body mass index (BMI) was carried out in a total of 225 patients, of whom 125 were men and 100 women. Analysis of BMI by sex found that normal weight in men was observed in 17.6% and in women—in 15.0% of cases. However, being overweight, i.e., BMI values from 25 to 30 kg/m^2 were recorded in men much more often than in women (52.8 and 37.0%, respectively, men and women, p = 0.001 и $\chi2$ = 10,573). Obesity of varying severity, in contrast, was more often observed in women than in men (**Table 1**). This was confirmed during the correlation analysis (**Figure 2**).

Thus, depending on gender, it was found that ACS/AMI was more often recorded in men, amounting to 54.1%; the incidence of ACS/AMI among women was 45.9%. In the age aspect, men with ACS/AMI were younger than women, and in terms of weight characteristics, obesity of various severity prevailed among women (48.0% in women vs. 29.6% in men, p = 0.007).

According to anamnestic data, postponed cardiovascular catastrophes were more often observed in males. Namely, the transferred myocardial infarction (TMI) was noted by men 1.8 times more often than women (p = 0.0000 и $\chi2$ = 14,282); the

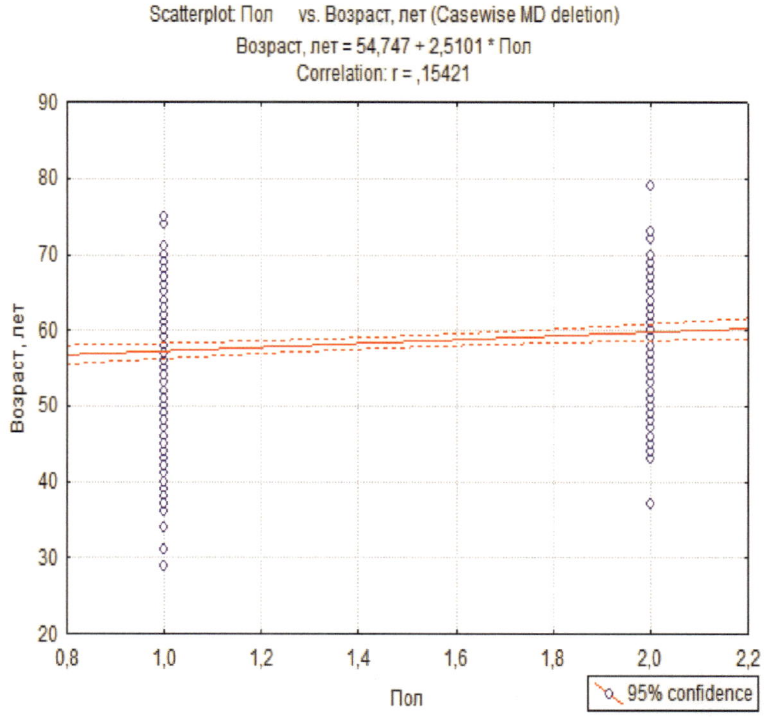

Figure 1.
Graph of correlation between gender and age of patients. p = 0.001; r = 0.154; t = 3.277. On the X-axis, the numeral "1"—male gender, and the numeral "2"—female gender; Y-axis, age of patients in years.

Indicator	Men (n = 243)	Women (n = 206)	p	χ2
Age, years	57.3 ± 8.6	59.8 ± 7.3	**0.001**	
Weight, kg	83.5 ± 11.2	79.2 ± 14.2	**0.012**	
Height, cm	171.7 ± 5.2	162.9 ± 6.1	**0.000**	
BMI, kg/m^2	28.4 ± 3.7	29.7 ± 4.6	**0.020**	
BMI measurement carried out, n (%)	**125 (51.4%)**	**100 (48.5%)**		
Normal weight, %	17.6	15.0	0.732	0.117
Excess weight (BMI = 25.1–30.0 kg/m^2), %	52.8	37.0	**0.026**	**4.969**
Obesity 1 degree (BMI = 30.1–35.0 kg/m^2), %	26.4	35.0	0.211	1.562
Obesity of 2 degrees, (BMI = 35.1–40.0 kg/m^2), %	2.4	10.0	**0.032**	4.581
Obesity of 3 degrees, (BMI ≥ 40.1 kg/m^2), %	0.8	3.0	0.458	0.550

Notes: n, the number of patients; p and χ2, significance of differences between groups; BMI, body mass index

Table 1.
Anthropometric characteristics of patients.

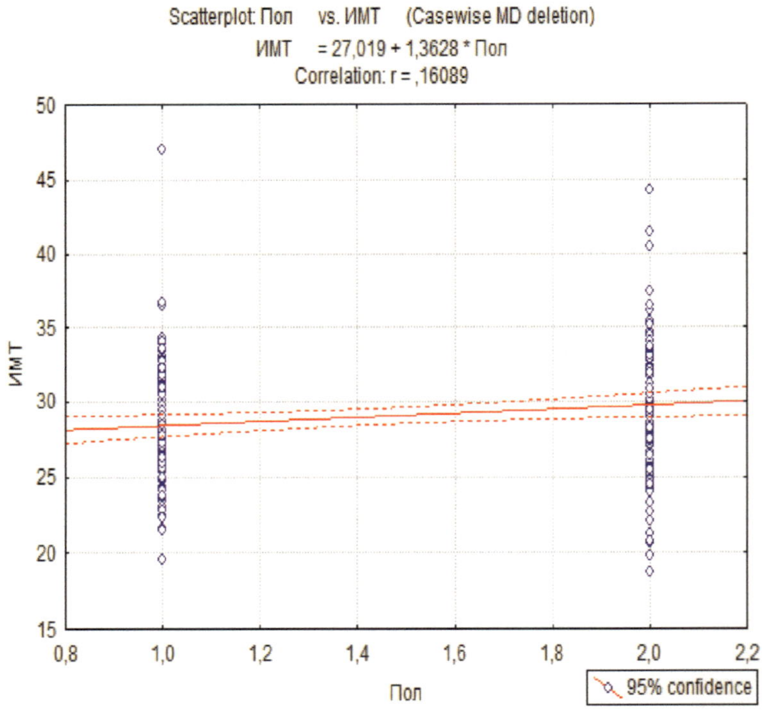

Figure 2.
Graph of correlation between gender and BMI of patients. p = 0.015; r = 0.161; t = 2.434. On the X-axis: The numeral "1"—male gender and the numeral "2"—female gender; Y-axis: BMI, body mass index in kg/m^2.

presence of a stroke in men was 1.7% more than in the female group; percutaneous coronary interventions (PCI) or coronary artery bypass surgery (CABG) in men was 11.5%, which was 3.3% more than in women (**Figure 3**).

The average age of women with TMI was 61.5 ± 7.8 years and of men = 58.4 ± 8.4 years (p = 0.041); on the contrary, the age of women with stroke was 59.6 ± 9.5 years and for men = 61.3 ± 7.1 years (p = 0.204).

The age of persons with cardiac surgery did not depend on any gender dependency: for women = 57.7 ± 7.1 years and for men = 58.6 ± 5.6 years (p = 0.246). Despite the fact that men with a history of TMI were younger, nevertheless, they were more likely to have stenotic contractions of ≥50%; however, revealed differences did not reach significance level.

The analysis of RFs is presented in **Figure 3**, from which it is clear that smoking, hypertension, and hypercholesterolemia (HChE) prevailed among men. In women, the main RFs were disorders of both carbohydrate and lipid metabolisms, hypertension, and obesity. The difference in RFs—smoking, impaired carbohydrate metabolism, and obesity—reached a statistically significant level (**Figure 4**). However, the total component of the RFs for the averaged value in women was less than in men: the average number of RFs in men = 3.6 ± 1.2 and in women = 2.4 ± 1.1 (p = 0.0000).

Thus, with ACS/AMI, gender-independent RFs turned out to be AH and HChE and gender-related—smoking (for men) and carbohydrate metabolism disorders and obesity (for women). The transferred of cardiovascular accidents was prerogative of males, while age was a controversial point in the development of this or that damage (TMI occurred in younger men and stroke in older men, compared to women).

The next stage of the study was an assessment of the patients' adherence to therapy, depending on gender. From these positions, there were no statistically significant differences between the groups. The average number of medications taken per day among men was 2.2 ± 1.7 per person and among women = 2.2 ± 1.6, respectively (p = 1.000). The substantive aspect of conservative therapy is presented in **Figure 5**, from which it can be seen that both men and women had approximately the same proportions for the main groups of drugs taken, but the difference did not reach significance level.

However, when calculating quantitative values, it was found that, in general, the female population turned out to be more committed to pharmacotherapy than the male population (the number of committed women was 80.6% against men = 75.7%, p = 0.261, and $\chi 2$ = 1.264). At the same time, the women's group prevailed in taking

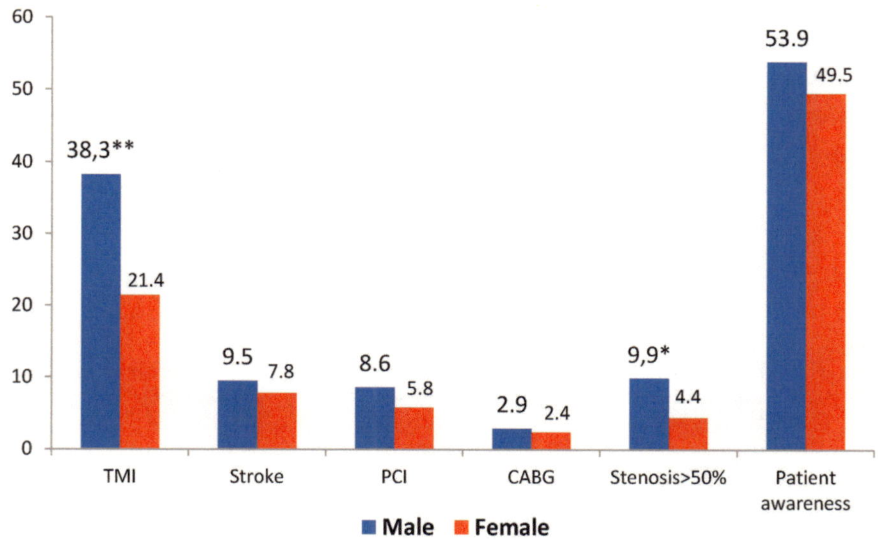

Figure 3.
*Anamnestic patient characteristics. Note: *significance of differences between groups at p < 0.05; **significance of differences between groups at p < 0.001; TMI, transferred myocardial infarction; PCI, percutaneous coronary intervention; CABG, coronary artery bypass grafting; presence of stenosis ≥ 50%; patient awareness of the presence of a cardiovascular pathology; data are presented in percentage.*

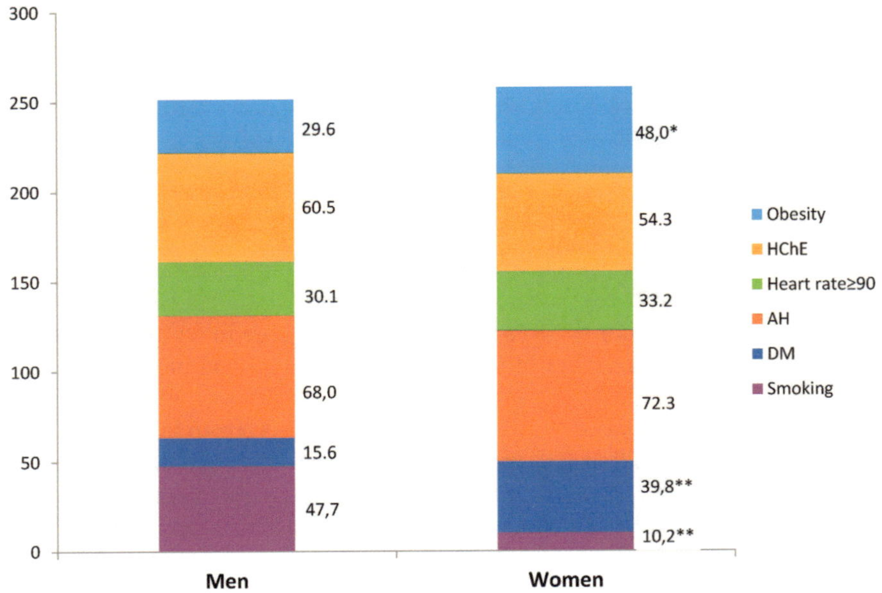

Figure 4.
*Risk factors by gender. Note: Data are presented in percentage; **significance of differences between groups with* $p < 0.001$ *and *a tendency to significance of differences between groups* ($p = 0.057$).

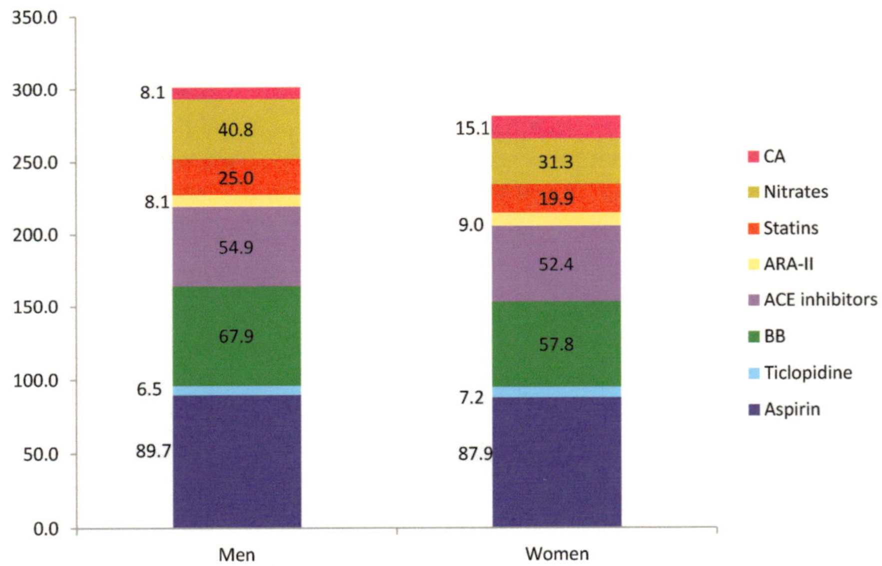

Figure 5.
The main groups of medications taken, depending on gender. Note: the data are presented in percentage, all $p > 0.05$; *ARA-II, angiotensin receptor antagonists-II; CA, calcium antagonists; BB, beta blockers.*

from 1 to 3 medicines per day, men's—from 4 or more pharmaceuticals per day, but the difference did not reach the level of confidence (**Table 2**).

A correlation analysis revealed that adherence to therapy increases with age, regardless of gender (**Figure 6**).

Thus, this fragment of the study showed that women's adherence to therapy was slightly higher than that of men; men were prone to taking more drugs, although the proportional ratio between the groups of drugs taken was not significantly

The number of medications taken per day	Men (n = 184)	Women (n = 166)	p	χ2
1 drug, %	17.4	20.5	0.548	0.362
2 drugs, %	20.6	22.3	0.809	0.059
3 drugs, %	26.1	29.5	0.551	0.356
4 drugs, %	23.9	19.9	0.435	0.609
5 drugs, %	9.8	6.6	0.381	0.766
6 and more drugs, %	2.2	1.2	0.776	0.081

Table 2.
Distribution of patients according to the daily ration of medications among men and women.

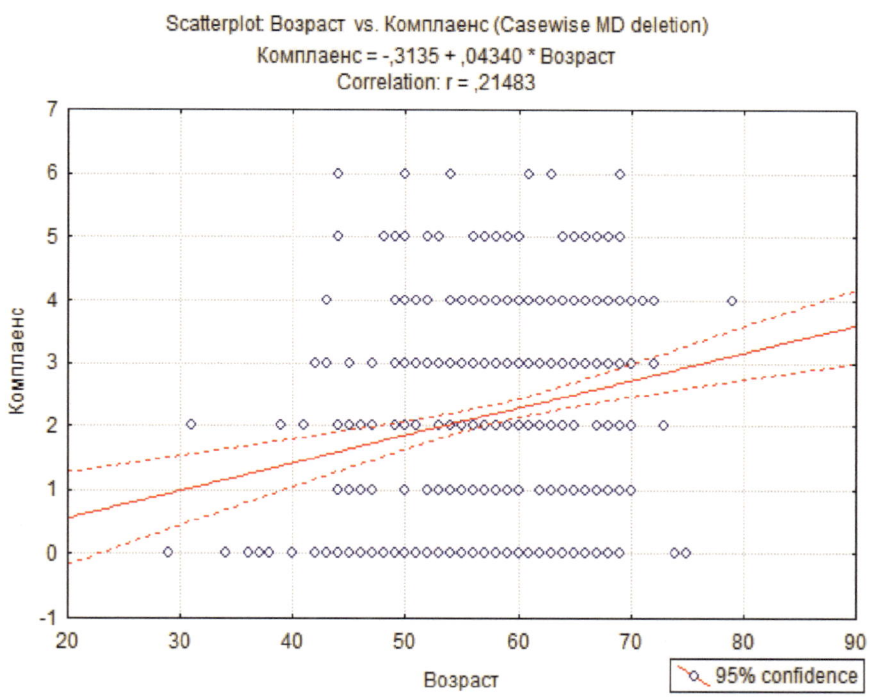

Figure 6.
Graph of correlation between age of patients and adherence to therapy. p = 0.000; r = 0.214; t = 4619. On the X-axis, age in years; on the Y-axis, the number of drugs taken per day.

different between men and women. However, a direct correlation was found between the age of the respondents and the number of medications taken per day.

2.3 The relationship of arterial hypertension with acute coronary events (a fragment of the study "RACSMI-Uz")

To assess the effect of hypertension, two groups were formed: group 1—47 respondents without hypertension (control group) and group 2—385 people with the presence of hypertension with varying severity. The groups were comparable in age and sex, as well as height-weight parameters. The distribution of individuals according to BMI established that the number of patients with overweight in the group with AH was significantly higher than in the control group ($p = 0.019$; $\chi2 = 5.520$), and the number of patients with AH and normal weight was almost two times less than in the control group (**Table 3**).

Indicators	Group 1 (control) n = 47	Group 2 (with the presence of AH) n = 385	p	χ2
Age, years	57.1 ± 9.8	58.6 ± 7.9	0.233	
Number of men, %	59.6%	53.9%		
Weight, kg	80.7 ± 16.6	81.7 ± 12.4	0.617	
Height, cm	168.4 ± 4.8	167.8 ± 7.3	0.583	
BMI, kg/m^2	28.5 ± 5.9	29.1 ± 4.1	0.370	
Normal weight, %	29.8	15.1	0.019	5.520
Obesity 1 degree, %	36.2	46.2	0.249	1.331
Obesity 2 degree, %	25.5	37.1	0.160	1.976
Obesity 3 degree, %	8.5	1.6	0.013	6.143

Notes: n, number of patients; AH, arterial hypertension; %, percentage of patients with this symptom; BMI, body mass index

Table 3.
Comparative characteristics of patient growth and weight indicators depending on the presence of arterial hypertension.

Analysis of anamnestic data showed that in group 2, individuals with myocardial infarction prevailed (33.2 and 8.5%, respectively, in groups 2 and 1; p = 0.000 and χ2 = 10.941). Also, hypertension was significantly more frequently accompanied by the development of chronic heart failure (53.3 and 23.4%, respectively, in groups 2 and 1; p = 0.000 and χ2 = 13.751). Patients with hypertension who underwent PCI or CABG were noted in 7.3 and 3.1% of cases, while in the control group, the corresponding figures were 8.5 and 0% (p = 0,110 и χ2 = 2554). The presence of stenoses >50% in the coronary vessels in the first group was detected in 4.3% of patients and in the second group—in 7.8% of the respondents (p = 0.562 и χ2 = 0.225). An individual conversation awareness of patients of acute coronary disease has been established in 53.5% of patients with hypertension and 38.3%—in the control group (p = 0.069; χ2 = 3.295). Analysis of bad habits did not reveal significant differences between groups. The number of nonsmokers among patients with hypertension was 59.5% and in the comparison group—55.3%. The number of smokers in group 2 was 24.1 and 25.5% in group 1; the number of people who stop smoking in group 2 was 16.4% and in 1 group—19.2%.

The clinical characteristics included in this fragment of patients showed that the average values of heart rate (HR) in both compared groups practically did not differ; however, HR > 80 beats/min among patients with AH was observed in 49.9% of cases, which is 1, five times more than in people without AH (**Table 4**).

Of the concomitant nosologies, the presence of type 2 diabetes mellitus (DM) among control group patients occurred in 4.3% and among patients with hypertension—in 34.8% of patients, while the average blood glucose level in group 1 was 5.8 ± 2.6 mmol/L and in group 2 = 6.3 ± 2.9 mmol/L (p = 0.260). Evaluation of the blood glucose level only in patients with DM showed that in the group with hypertension, this indicator was equal to 8.4 ± 3.5 mmol/L, which was 0.7 mmol/L higher than in the first group (p = 0.194).

Significant, but somewhat paradoxical, differences were found in the evaluation of blood lipid spectrum. Namely, the number of patients with hypercholesterolemia was 1.5 times higher among patients of the first group, i.e., without hypertension, which was confirmed by digital indicators in blood tests. However, the average level of triglycerides among respondents without AH was 1.5 times lower than in the comparison group (**Table 5**).

Indicators	Group 1 (control) n = 47	Group 2 (with the presence of AH) n = 385	p	χ2
HR > 80 beats/min	34.1	49.9	0.058	3.593
Average HR, beats/min	80.8 ± 16.7	84.6 ± 18.2	0.174	
The average HR in patients with HR > 80 beats/min	97.7 ± 15.8	96.3 ± 17.4	0.599	
Mean SBP, mm Hg	115.9 ± 10.1	143.8 ± 27.7	**0.000**	
Mean DBP, mm Hg	75.1 ± 9.3	87.1 ± 13.8	**0.000**	

Notes: n, the number of patients; SBP and DBP, systolic and diastolic blood pressure

Table 4.
Comparative characteristics of hemodynamic parameters of patients depending on the presence of arterial hypertension.

Indicators	Group 1 (control) n = 47	Group 2 (with the presence of AH) n = 385	p	χ2
The number of patients with normal levels of TCh	19.2%	46.2%	**0.000**	11.438
The average level of TCh, mg/dL	205.6 ± 46.6	156.7 ± 92.9	**0.000**	
The average level of TCh in patients with HChE	221.25 ± 36.1	205.1 ± 82.6	0.186	
The number of patients with HChE	80.8%	53.8%	**0.000**	11.438
The average level of TG, mg/dL	143.1 ± 80.7	211.7 ± 186.2	**0.013**	

Notes: n, the number of patients; TCh, total cholesterol; HChE, hypercholesterolemia; TG, triglycerides

Table 5.
Lipid blood spectrum of the compared patient groups.

Analysis of the main ECG changes in ACS/AMI in the studied patient groups revealed that for individuals with hypertension, the most characteristic are ST-segment depression (35.6% in 2 g and 25.5% in 1 g; p = 0.228; χ2 = 1.455) and inversion of the T-wave without ST-displacement (16.3% in 2g and 8.5% in 1g; p = 0.234; χ2 = 1.418), while ST-elevation was observed <15% of cases (**Figure** 7).

The distribution of patients of group 2 according to the level of BP showed that optimal, normal, and high-normal BP occurred in 37.7% of cases, and in the remaining 62.3%, there was AH of varying severity (**Figure** 8). The distribution of optimal, normal, and high-normal levels of BP in the second group is probably due to received antihypertensive therapy.

An in-depth comparative assessment of the clinical and functional parameters of patients depending on the degree of AH showed that in patients with grade 2 hypertension, the number of patients with DM was much higher than among patients with grade 1 hypertension or grade 3 hypertension, but the average blood glucose level was not a significant difference. It was also found that over 50% of patients with AH, regardless of its degree, were characterized by elevated heart rate.

However, the correlation analysis did not reveal the relationship between HR and BP values (p = 0.564; t = −0.576). In addition, patients with hypertension had elevated levels of blood triglycerides, especially those with hypertension first and third degree (p = 0.0000); however, indicators of total cholesterol were lower than

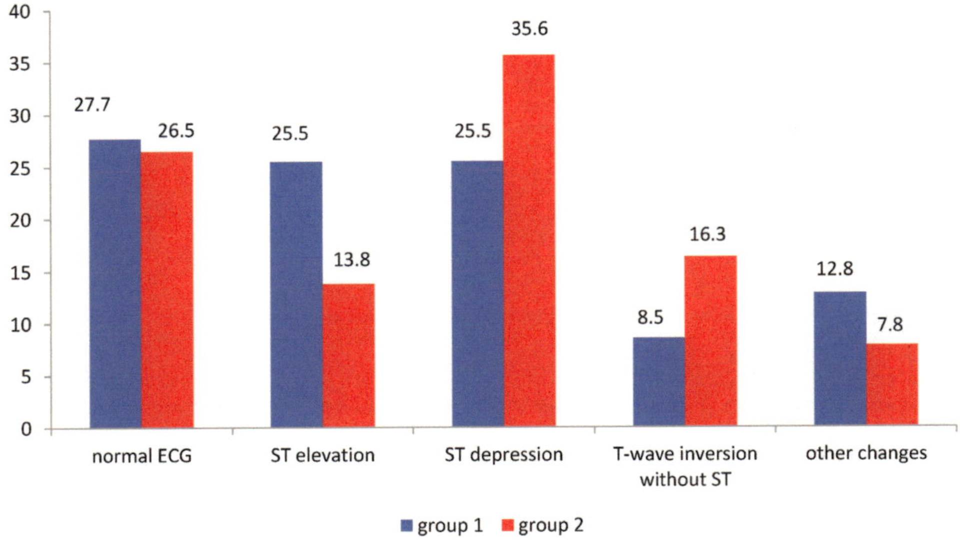

Figure 7.
The occurrence of ECG changes in the compared groups of patients (%).

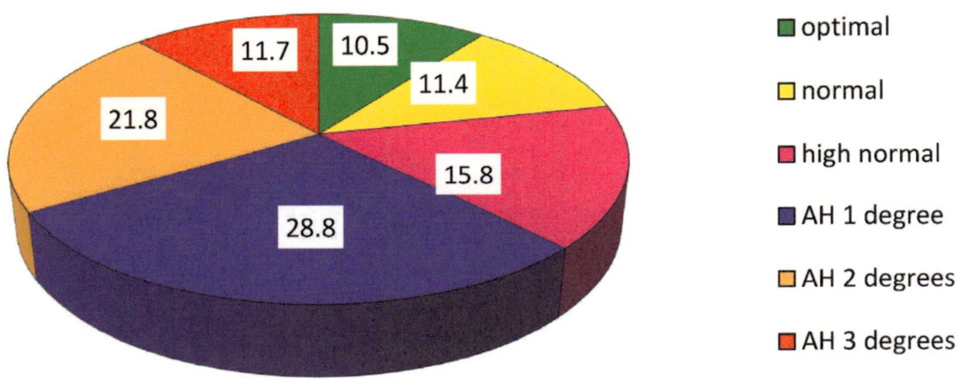

Figure 8.
Distribution of patients in group 2 by blood pressure levels.

in the control group. When comparing the lipid spectrum with the blood pressure numbers, no correlation dependence was found. According to ECG parameters, there were no significant differences in the analyzed patients; with the exception of ST-elevation, the phenomenon of which was less frequently observed among respondents with AH 2 degree (**Table 6**).

The evaluation of the treatment of patients with AH, regardless of its severity, showed that all patients in this category took on average 2.4 ± 1.6 drugs, which was two times higher than in the control group; however, antihypertensive drugs such as BB and ACE inhibitors among people with AH were used much more often than in the control group (**Table** 7).

2.4 Comparative analysis of patients with acute coronary events depending on the presence/absence of diabetes mellitus (data from the "RACSMI-Uz" registry)

To assess the impact of DM, two groups were identified: group 1, 207 respondents without diabetes (control group), and group 2, 159 people with DM, of which

Indicators	Control group (n = 47)	Patients with AH 1 (n = 105)	Patients with AH 2 (n = 79)	Patients with AH 3 (n = 42)
Age, years	57.1 ± 9.8	58.8 ± 7.9	60.2 ± 6.6*	58.9 ± 7.3
Number of men, % of patients	59.6	55.2	41.8	57.1
BMI, kg/m2	28.5 ± 5.9	29.1 ± 3.8	27.9 ± 3.1	30.3 ± 4.9
DM, % of patients	4.3	29.5*	38**	30.9*
The average level of blood glucose, mmol/L	5.8 ± 2.6	6.1 ± 2.4	6.1 ± 2.2	6.0 ± 2.4
HR > 80 beats/min, % of patients	34.1	58.1*	55.7*	59.5*
Average HR, beats/min	80.8 ± 16.7	84.3 ± 13.7	85.5 ± 16.4	84.8 ± 12.7
Characteristics of BP				
Mean SBP, mm Hg	115.9 ± 10.1	143.7 ± 4.9**	162.2 ± 4.1**	193.8 ± 21.3**
Average DBP, mm Hg	75.1 ± 9.3	89.1 ± 7.0**	95.9 ± 7.3**	101.7 ± 17.3**
The average level of TCh, mg/dL	205.6 ± 46.6	177.3 ± 82.5*	1977 ± 45.2	167.3 ± 31.5**
The average level of TG, mg/dL	146.1 ± 80.7	222.5 ± 188.7*	160.1 ± 53.4	232.3 ± 45.3**
ECG changes				
Normal ECG, %	27.7	27.6	24.1	28.6
Elevation ST, %	25.5	12.4	6.3*	14.3
Depression ST, %	25.5	42.9	40.5	40.5
Inversion of the T-wave without ST, %	8.5	14.3	20.2	9.5
Other changes	12.8	2.8%*	8.9	7.1
Commitment to therapy				
The average number of medications taken	1.2 ± 1.5	2.4 ± 1.5**	2.4 ± 1.6**	2.7 ± 1.7**
BB, %	27.7	53.3*	48.1*	54.8*
ACE inhibitors/ARA, %	17.0/0	46.7/8.6**	51.9/3.8*	57.1/7.1**
Calcium antagonists	6.4	11.4	6.3	14.3
Aspirin	40.4	74.3**	74.7**	80.9**
Nitrates	17.0	22.9	31.6	47.6*
Statins	10.6	19.1	20.2	11.9

**significance of differences in comparison with the control group at p < 0.05*
***the significance of differences in comparison with the control group at p < 0.001Notes: OH, total cholesterol; TG, triglycerides; BB, β-blockers; ACE inhibitors, angiotensin-converting enzyme inhibitors; ARA, angiotensin II receptor antagonists.*

Table 6.
Comparative analysis of clinical and functional parameters depending on the degree of hypertension.

41.5% had diabetes compensated by diet, 38.4% had diabetes compensated by taking hypoglycemic drug tablets, 6.9% had diabetes compensated by insulin intake, and 13.2% had newly diagnosed type 2 diabetes.

Indicator	Group 1 without DM (n = 207)	Group 2 with DM (n = 159)	p	χ2
Number of men, %	62.3	46.5	**0.004**	**8.435**
Number of women, %	37.7	53.5		
The average age of men, years	57.1 ± 8.9	58.7 ± 8.1	0.208	
The average age of women, years	58.6 ± 7.7	61.2 ± 6.9*	**0.024**	
Weight, kg	80.1 ± 11.2	83.8 ± 13.5	**0.004**	
Height, cm	168.4 ± 6.6	168.7 ± 6.9	0.673	
BMI, kg/m^2	28.2 ± 3.5	30.2 ± 4.6	**0.000**	
Obesity, n (%)	80.7	87.4	0.113	2.513
Normal weight (BMI = 18–24.9 kg/m^2), %	19.3	12.6		
Excess weight (BMI = 25–29.9 kg/m^2), %	52.2	35.2	**0.002**	**9.777**
Obesity grade (BMI = 30–34.9 kg/m^2), %	25.6	39.6	**0.006**	**7.529**
Obesity grade 2 (BMI = 35–39.9 kg/m^2), %	2.9	8.8	**0.020**	**5.450**
Obesity grade 3 (BMI ≥40 kg/m^2), %	0	3.8	**0.016**	**5.774**

**p = 0.036 in the intragroup comparison of the average age of men and women*
Note: BMI, body mass index; n, the number of patients; DM, diabetes mellitus

Table 7.
Gender-anthropometric characteristics of compared groups of patients.

The study found that patients in group 2 were much older than patients in group 1 (mean age of patients in group 1 = 57.7 ± 8.5 years and in group 2 = 60.1 ± 7.6 years; p = 0.005). The age difference was due to the predominance of young people in group 1. Namely, the category of ≤45 years in group 1 was 9.7%, and in group 2–3.8% (p = 0.049 и χ2 = 3874) of respondents (**Figure 9**).

On the contrary, in group 2 the number of patients older than 66 years was greater than in the comparison group (28.9 vs. 21.7%, p = 0.170 и χ2 = 1880).

The average age of men was younger than the average age of women, regardless of the presence or absence of diabetes. This difference in group 2 reaches the level of confidence (**Table 7**). Correlation analysis between age and the presence of DM has established a direct relationship (**Figure 10**).

Gender-anthropometric characteristics of patients are presented in **Table 7**, from which it can be seen that in group 2, the number of women was greater than in group 1, and the weight characteristics of patients in group 2 exceeded those in patients of the comparison group. A more detailed analysis found that among persons with DM, obesity of varying severity was more common (52.2 vs. 28.5%, respectively, in groups 2 and 1; p = 0.000 и χ2 = 20,284).

A correlation analysis revealed a direct relationship between blood glucose and BMI, as well as between gender and diabetes, while in the latter case, the correlation reached a statistically significant level (**Figures 11** and **12**).

BP was measured in 94.7% of respondents in the first group and in 95.6% in the second group: a total of 348 patients. The mean figures of both systolic and diastolic BP were comparable between the groups, as well as the quantitative components of the main gradations of BP. The presence of AH in individuals of group 1 was in 48.3% of cases, and in group 2—in 49.7% of cases (**Table 8**). When carrying out the correlation analysis, we did not reveal any relationship between the blood glucose level and the BP values.

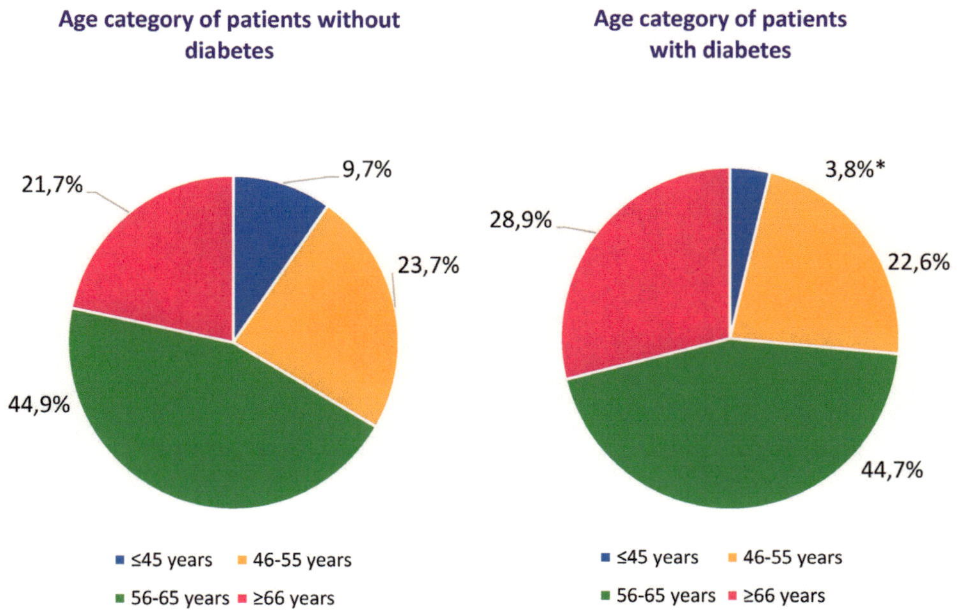

Figure 9.
*The distribution of patients by age. *significance of differences between groups at p < 0.05.*

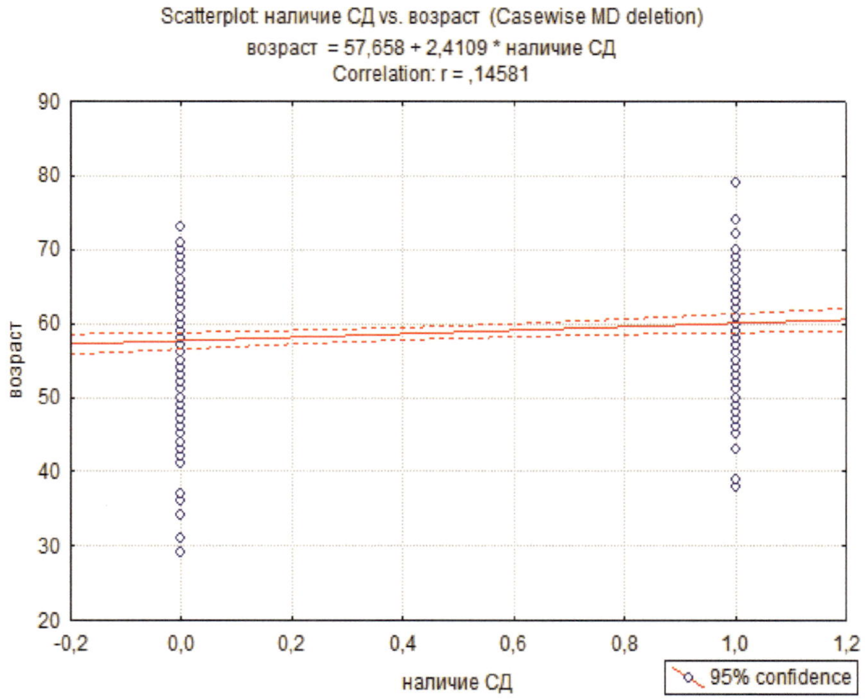

Figure 10.
Graph of correlation between the presence of diabetes and age of patients. p = 0.005; t = 2781; r = 0.145. On the X-axis, "0" is the absence of SD and "1" is the presence of SD; on the Y-axis, age of patients in years.

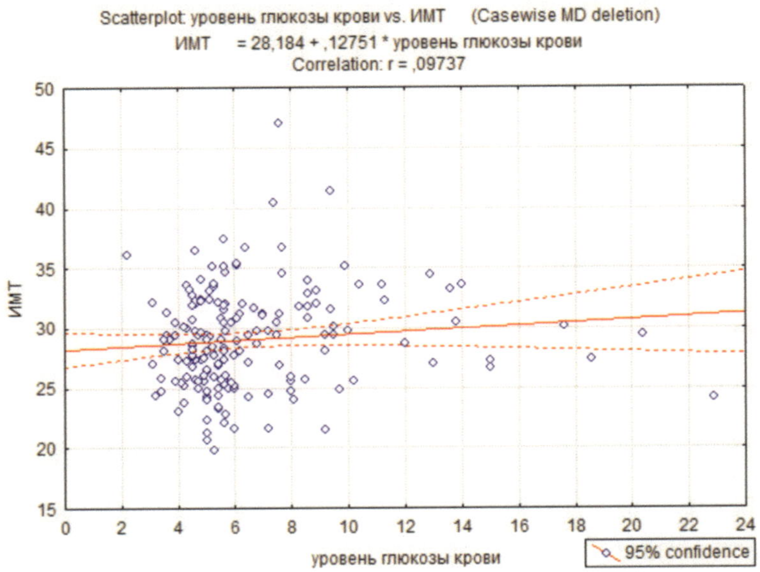

Figure 11.
The graph of the correlation between the level of blood glucose (mmol/L): X-axis and body mass index (kg/m²); Y-axis, p = 0.202; t = 1.279; r = 0.097.

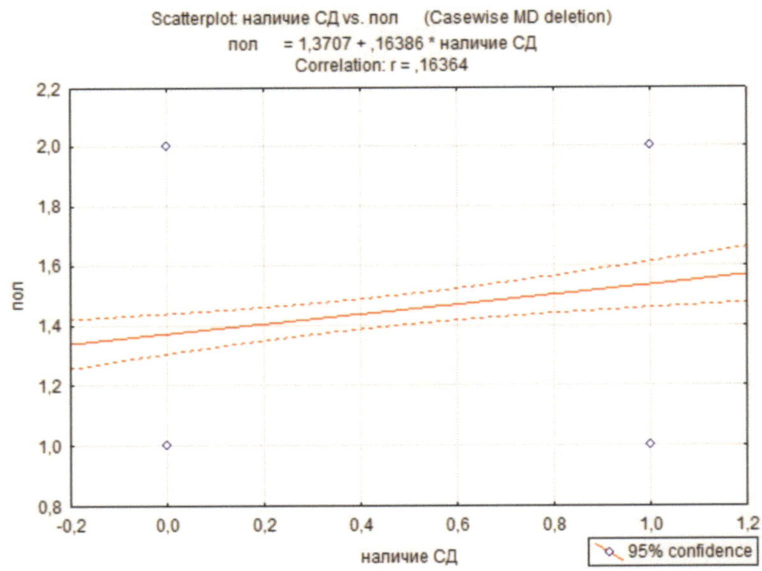

Figure 12.
Graph of correlation between the presence of DM and gender. p = 0.001; t = 3.156; r = 0.163. On the X-axis, "0" is the absence of DM and "1" is the presence of DM; on the Y-axis, "1" men and "2" women.

Analysis of lipid metabolism was carried out in 1/5 of the subjects, 40 of them from group 1 and 36 from group 2. In this aspect, it was found that the levels of total cholesterol in group 1 = 187.8 ± 51.5 mg/dL and in group 2 = 199.1 ± 47.8 mg/dL (p = 0.326). The number of patients with total cholesterol over 180 mg/dL in the first group was 55.0% and in the second group—61.1% of patients, while the average level of total blood cholesterol in the first group = 222.1 ± 40.2 mg/dL and in group 2 = 224.1 ± 43.6 mg/dL (p = 0.514).

Indicator	Group 1 without DM (n = 196)	Group 2 with DM (n = 152)	p	$\chi 2$
Mean SBP, mm Hg	138.8 ± 29.4	138.3 ± 28.4	0.873	
Mean DBP, mm Hg	85.0 ± 15.9	83.9 ± 14.0	0.501	
Optimal BP < 120 mm Hg, %	15.8	19.7	0.417	0.659
Normal BP, 120–129 mm Hg, %	15.3	15.1	0.916	0.011
High-normal BP, 130–139 mm Hg, %	17.9	13.2	0.297	1.090
AH-1 degree, 140–159 mm Hg, %	25.5	21.7	0.485	0.487
AH-2 degrees, 160–179 mm Hg, %	15.8	20.4	0.334	0.933
AH-3 degrees, ≥180 mm.rt.st., %	9.7	9.9	0.898	0.016

Notes: n, the number of patients; SBP/DBP, systolic/diastolic blood pressure; DM, diabetes mellitus; AH, arterial hypertension

Table 8.
Blood pressure indicators depending on the presence or absence of diabetes.

Analysis of blood triglyceride levels revealed a clear prevalence of this indicator in patients with diabetes (159.8 ± 83.1 mg/dL in the first group and 261.9 ± 217.85 mg/dL in the second group, p = 0.015). The number of patients with hypertriglyceridemia in group 1 was 17.5% and in group 2—41.7% of patients (p = 0.054; $\chi 2$ = 3.701), while the content of blood triglycerides in group 1 = 283.0 ± 90.1 mg/dL for and in group 2 = 426.2 ± 222.6 mg/dL (p = 0.120). When carrying out the correlation analysis, a directly proportional relationship was established; i.e., an increase in blood glucose levels is directly correlated with an increase in blood triglyceride levels, while the dependence was not so pronounced with total cholesterol (**Figures 13** and **14**). From the above, it follows that the presence of diabetes is associated with dyslipidemia, in particular with hypertriglyceridemia.

From anamnestic data, it was found that chronic heart failure was more often observed among patients of group 2 (56.0 vs. 45.4% of cases in groups 2 and 1, respectively, p = 0.058, $\chi 2$ = 3.603). 34.8% in the first group and 31.4% of patients in the second group were indicated on the transferred AMI in the anamnesis. Previously, PCI/CABG was observed in 9.2 and 3.4% of respondents in group 1 and 9.4 and 1.9% of persons in group 2. However, stenosis >50% was more common in patients with diabetes than in the comparison group (78.9% in group 1 and 93.3% in group 2, p = 0.005, $\chi 2$ = 7.905).

One of the fragments of the study was the analysis of thrombolytic therapy (TLT). From this perspective, it was found that TLT in group 1 was performed in 54.1% and in group 2 in 59.1% of patients. At the same time, the success of the TLT procedure in group 1 was 62.5% and in group 2—60.6%. This was also confirmed during the correlation analysis, which showed that the blood glucose level did not affect the success of the TLT procedure (p = 0.944; t = 0.069; r = 0.005). However, a more detailed analysis found that among patients of group 2, the form of DM is of considerable importance when conducting TLT. **Figure 15** presents a graph of the correlation dependence between various forms of DM and the success of TLT. As can be seen in **Figure 15**, the TLT procedure was more successful in patients who are on glucose-lowering drugs, including insulin therapy, and in patients with newly diagnosed forms of the disease (**Figure 15**).

Thus, in patients with ACS/AMI, comorbid with diabetes, the success of thrombolysis was directly dependent on the form of diabetes and ongoing antidiabetic therapy.

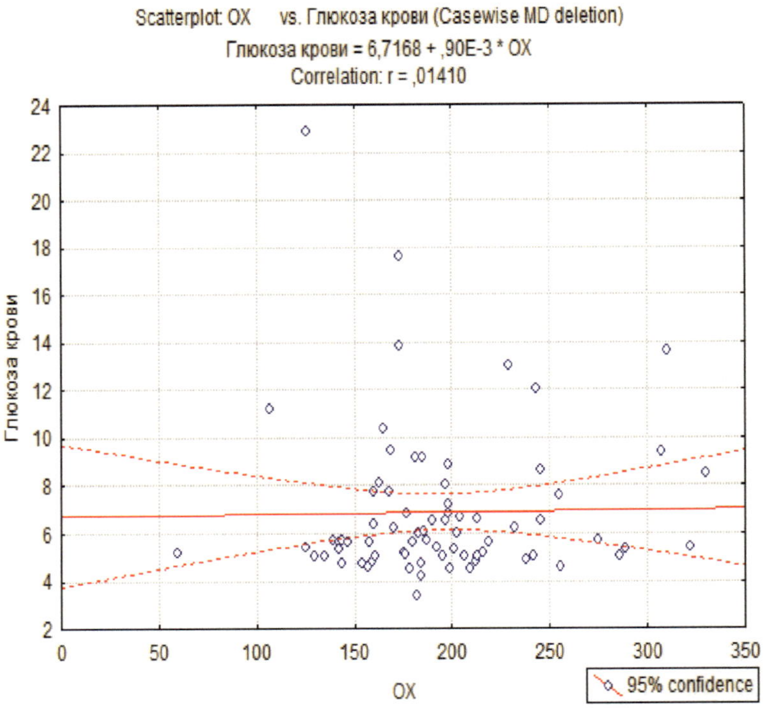

Figure 13.
The graph of the correlation between the level of blood glucose and total cholesterol (n = 76). p = 0.905; t = 0.119; r = 0.014; X-axis, total cholesterol values; Y-axis, blood glucose values.

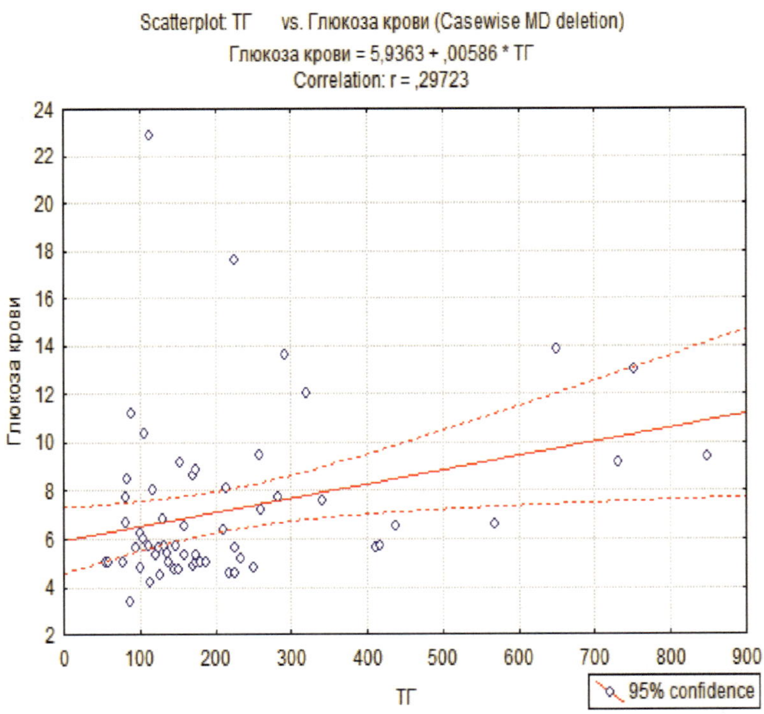

Figure 14.
The graph of the correlation between the level of blood glucose and triglycerides (n = 76). p = 0.021; t = 2.371; r = 0,279. On the X-axis, the values of triglycerides; Y-axis, blood glucose values.

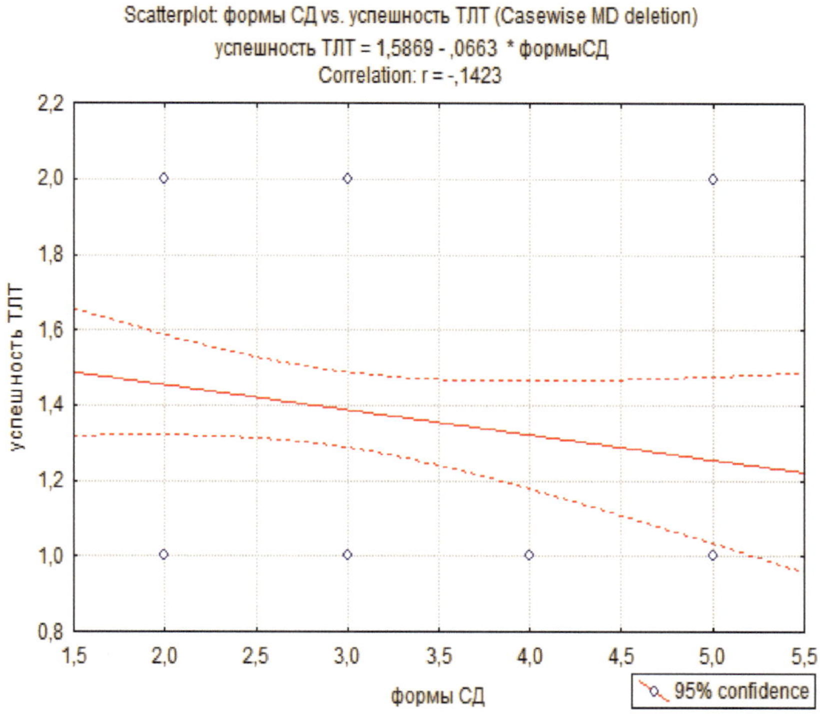

Figure 15.
Graph of correlation between various forms of diabetes and the success of the TLT procedure. $p = 0.171$; $t = -1.3784$ $r = -0.142$; *Notes: On the X-axis, the number "2," DM compensated by diet; the number "3," DM compensated by the intake of tablets medications; the number "4," DM compensated by insulin; and the number "5," the first revealed diabetes; on the Y-axis, numeral "1," a successful thrombolytic therapy (TLT), and the numeral "2," unsuccessful TLT.*

2.5 Discussion of the results of the study "RACSMI-Uz"

Gender is a very significant factor in the occurrence and course of AMI. Men get sick much more often than women, especially at young and middle ages, but with increasing age, these differences disappear. The cause of female immunity to AMI at a young age is due to the subtleties of the hormonal system of the body of women, with a significant role belongs to an increased amount of estrogen. This is the main hormone of the female reproductive system, taking an active part in the reproductive function. Estrogen in the female body performs a number of functions, one of which is the dilation of the heart's own blood vessels, which contributes to leaching of sclerotic plaques and prolonging the normal functioning of the myocardium [13]. After menopause, the hormonal system of the female body significantly changes its work, and the content of estrogen in the blood decreases. This leads to a violation of the protection of coronary vessels from harmful influences and the development of CHD [13]. The results of our register revealed that women with ACS/AMI were older than men, and, for the most part, age over 50 years prevailed. Unfortunately, in the map-register used by us, there were no questions concerning the state of health of the female body; therefore, we cannot judge the hormonal status of the analyzed female population. However, the identified age limit—over 50 years old—can probably be considered as evidence of the menopausal period of women included in this register.

Most of the generally recognized RFs of CVD are common for men and women; however, the accumulated scientific data to date indicate the presence of certain features of the manifestation of RF in the female population [14–16]. In our registry, the majority of patients had combined cardiac pathology, with the most frequent option being a combination of CHD and AH (over 80% of patients).

The study found that the average level of triglycerides in respondents with hypertension was 1.5 times higher than in the comparison group. According to scientific information sources, an increased level of triglycerides is observed in those who already have high levels of low-density lipoproteins and low levels of high-density lipoproteins in the blood; are obese; have type 2 diabetes, decreased thyroid function, and neurotic syndrome; and consume excessive amounts of alcohol. It is completely natural to ask whether triglycerides are related to an increased cardiovascular risk in these patients or whether they simply reflect metabolic disturbances. The final answer to the question about the participation of triglycerides in the process of atherosclerotic vascular lesion has not yet been received. It is assumed that an increase in triglycerides reflects an increased content of atherogenic lipid particles, such as intermediate density lipoproteins and very low-density lipoproteins, which, among other things, cause and maintain inflammation of the vascular wall [17]. Probably, this is the explanation of the hypertriglyceridemia detected in our registry specifically in individuals with hypertension.

In the CREATE-ECLA study, 30-day mortality in patients with AMI with ST-elevation differed significantly depending on the glucose content in the blood and was 6.6% of patients with glycemia within the lower tertile and 14% of patients with glycemia within the upper tertile [18, 19]. According to the register of the RECORD, the presence of diabetes, as the FR of the development of ACS, occurred in 18.1% of respondents [20]. The results of our study "ROXIM-Uz" revealed that 34.8% of patients with hypertension had concomitant diabetes.

It is well-known that people who are overweight and obese have a higher risk of developing metabolic syndrome, type 2 diabetes, AH, and CHD [21]. Findings from epidemiological studies have repeatedly confirmed the strong positive relationship between obesity and the risk of developing DM. In our study, a similar trend is observed. In the group of patients with DM, the number of people with obesity of varying severity was 1.8 times greater than in the group of patients without diabetes.

One of the most important causes of high cardiovascular morbidity and mortality in patients with diabetes is the accelerated development of the atherosclerotic process [22]. In our study, it was found that stenosis >50% was more often detected in patients with diabetes (93.3%) than in the comparison group (78.9%). Endothelial dysfunction is the earliest stage in the development of adverse cardiovascular complications in patients with diabetes [23]. However, the relationship between diabetes and vascular pathology remains unclear.

Under conditions of hyperglycemia, there is an increased formation of the end products of glycation and their precursors, which leads to a change in the structure of blood proteins and the extracellular matrix, disrupting the function of nerve fibers. Levels of all previous glycolysis intermediates become elevated, which triggers alternative paths; glyceraldehyde-3-phosphate, glycerol, and methylglyoxal enter the pathway of protein kinase C and the end products of glycation, fructose-6-phosphate enters the hexosamine pathway, and glucose itself enters the polyol pathway. All the above pathological pathways for utilization of glucose and its metabolites cause diabetic complications and damage to the nervous tissue and the vascular wall (neuropathy and angiopathy) [24].

To verify the positive effect of insulin on the course of AMI in patients with diabetes, a diabetes, insulin, glucose infusion in acute myocardial infarction (DIGAMI) study was conducted, which showed that with the development of AMI in patients with diabetes, adding to therapy the glucose-insulin-potassium mixture followed by insulin therapy can reduce mortality after 1 and 3 years. [25, 26]. The direct correlation between the forms of diabetes and the success of TLT identified in our study is probably due to the fact that patients receiving hypoglycemic drugs, including insulin therapy, are characterized by relatively intact endothelial functionality and, thus, have a more favorable prognosis than patients, adhering to dietary recommendations only.

Numerous studies confirm the positive effect of treatment standards for treating one or the other diseases [27]. The results of our register showed that persons with ACS/AMI comorbid with AH are characterized by high adherence to therapy with β-blockers and ACE inhibitors; however, despite this, they still developed destabilization of CHD, probably due to, as mentioned above, the development of refractoriness to drug therapy.

In work Wang et al. [28] when analyzing 382 elderly patients from six Macau Medical Centers, China, the best adherence to therapy was observed in people over 65 years of age. A similar trend has occurred in our register. As for the predominance of women in the group of committed patients that we received during the course of work, this fact is confirmed by other researchers who show that women are more committed to treatment than men [29–31].

Thus, the register "RACSMI-Uz" conducted in the clinic conditions of the Republican Specialized Scientific Medical Center for Cardiology allowed obtaining objective data on the demographic, anamnestic, and clinical characteristics of patients with acute coronary pathology in only one of the districts of Tashkent city. The results obtained revealed both positive aspects in the treatment plan of this category of patients and established a number of issues that require further study.

3. Conclusions

ACS/AMI is more commonly reported in men. In the age aspect, men with ACS/AMI turned out to be younger than women, and in terms of weight characteristics, obesity of varying severity prevailed among women.

With ACS/AMI, gender-independent risk factors (RF) were hypertension and hypercholesterolemia GHS, and gender-related factors were smoking (for men) and carbohydrate metabolism disorders and obesity (for women). The history of cardiovascular catastrophes was prerogative of males, while age seemed to be a controversial point in the development of this or that damage (TMI occurred in younger men and stroke in older men compared with women).

Adherence to therapy in women was slightly higher than in men, although in a proportional ratio in the accepted groups of drugs, there were no significant differences between men and women. However, a direct correlation was found between the age of the respondents and the number of medications taken per day. Adherence to taking drugs in patients with ACS/AMI with comorbid hypertension was two times higher than among those without hypertension.

Arterial hypertension as a risk factor was recorded in 89% of patients with ACS/AMI, of which in 36.7% of cases hypertension was noted in history and in 52.3% of cases—hypertension of various severity occurred at the present time.

In ACS/AMI, concomitant comorbid conditions, such as obesity, previous myocardial infarction, chronic heart failure, and type 2 diabetes, were the prerogative of individuals with hypertension and, accordingly, were characterized by a large number of patients with stenotic >50% of the coronary arteries.

In ACS/AMI, the number of patients with heart rate > 80 beats/min among patients with AH was 1.5 times more than among those without it; however, when considering heart rate depending on the degree of AH, no significant differences were found.

The lipid spectrum of patients with ACS/AMI, comorbid with AH, was characterized by hypertriglyceridemia and relatively intact values of total blood cholesterol, while ST-segment depression and T-wave inversion were more often recorded on the ECG than the ST-elevation.

In patients with acute coronary events comorbid with DM, a direct correlation was observed with age, female sex, obesity, and hypertriglyceridemia; on the contrary, no dependence was found between the blood pressure figures and the blood glucose level.

In patients with ACS/AMI, in combination with DM, symptoms of chronic heart failure were observed much more often than in individuals without diabetes, which was probably due to a significantly higher incidence of diagnostically significant stenotic constriction in the coronary arteries.

In patients with ACS/AMI comorbid with DM, the success of thrombolysis was directly dependent on the form of diabetes and hypoglycemic therapy.

Acknowledgement

I express my gratitude to the employees of the register "RACSMI-Uz" who took part in the collection of information: Aminov A. A., Abidova D. E., Alieva Z. Kh., Mun O. R., Urinov O., and Mamarajapova D. A.

Also, on behalf of the participants of the "RACSMI-Uz" register, the staff of the Republican Specialized Scientific-Practical Medical Center for Cardiology of the Ministry of Health of the Republic of Uzbekistan expresses gratitude to the administrative and medical workers of the city clinical hospitals, family polyclinics and emergency medical care in Mirzo-Ulugbek district of Tashkent for their cooperation and assistance in conducting this project.

Conflict of interest

In the course of the "ROXIM-Uz" register, no conflicts of interest arose.

Abbreviations

ACS	acute coronary syndrome
AMI	acute myocardial infarction
ACE inhibitors	angiotensin-converting enzyme inhibitors
ARA	angiotensin II receptor antagonists
AH	arterial hypertension
BB	β-blockers
BP	blood pressure
beats/min	beats per minute
BMI	body mass index
CA	calcium antagonists
CVD	cardiovascular diseases
CABG	coronary artery bypass grafting
CHD	coronary heart disease
DM	diabetes mellitus
DBP	diastolic blood pressure
ECG	electrocardiogram
HR	heart rate

HChE	hypercholesterolemia
IDF	international diabetes federation
mm Hg	millimeters of mercury
PCI	percutaneous coronary intervention
TMI	transferred myocardial infarction
RACSMI-Uz	register of acute coronary syndrome and myocardial infarction in Uzbekistan
RF	risk factors for coronary artery disease
SBP	systolic blood pressure
TLT	thrombolytic therapy
TCh	total cholesterol
TG	triglycerides

Author details

Nagaeva Gulnora
Republican Specialized Scientific and Practical Medical Center of Cardiology, Tashkent, Uzbekistan

*Address all correspondence to: nagaeva.gulnora@mail.ru

References

[1] Fletcher RH, Fletcher SW. Clinical Epidemiology: The Essentials. Vol. 4th–xv. London: Lippincott Williams and Wilkins; 2005. 252p

[2] D'Agostino RB Sr, Vasan RS, Pencina MJ, Wolf PA, Cobain M, Massaro JM, et al. General cardiovascular risk profile for use in primary care: The Framingham heart study. Circulation. 2008;**117**(6):743-753

[3] Pencina MJ, D'Agostino RB Sr, Larson MG, Massaro JM, Vasan RS. Predicting the 30-year risk of cardiovascular disease: The Framingham heart study. Circulation. 2009;**119**(24): 3078-3084

[4] Gliklich RE, Dreyer NA, Leavy MB, editors. Registries for Evaluating Patient Outcomes: A User's Guide [Internet]. 3rd ed. US, Rockville (MD): Agency for Healthcare Research and Quality; Apr 2014. Report No.: 13(14)-EHC111. AHRQ Methods for Effective Health Care

[5] Ginzburg ML. Evaluation of the immediate and long-term results of treatment of patients with acute myocardial infarction within the register [Material doctoral dissertation]. Moscow; 2016. 211p. Available from: https://www.gnicpm.ru/data/files/dictionary/1547/158/DissertationGinzburgML.pdf

[6] Kronenberg GM, Mel-med S, Polonsky KS, Larsen PR. In: Dedova II, Melnichenko GA, editors. Diabetes and Carbohydrate Metabolism: Translation from English. Moscow, Russia: Reed Elsiver LLC; 2010. 448p

[7] Lorber D. Importance of cardiovascular disease risk with type 2 diabetes mellitus. Diabetes, Metabolic Syndrome and Obesity. 2014;**7**:169-183

[8] Donath MY, Shoelson SE. Type 2 diabetes as an inflammatory disease. Nature Reviews Immunology. 14 Jan 2011;**11**:98-107

[9] Ametov AS, Kurochkin IO, Zubkov AA. Diabetes mellitus and cardiovascular diseases. Russian Medical Journal. Endocrinology. 2014;**13**: 943-958

[10] ESC Congress 2018. Focus on Updated Recommendations for the Treatment of Hypertension. Available from: https://www.umj.com.ua/article/130071/esc-congress-2018-aktsent-na-obnovlennye-rekomendatsii-po-lecheniyu-arterialnoj-gipertenzii

[11] Repeated myocardial infarction of unspecified localization (I22.9). Version: Directory of Diseases MedElement. Available from: https://diseases.medelement.com/disease/3787

[12] Methods of diagnosis of myocardial infarction. Available from: https://serdce.biz/diagnostika/diagnostika-infarkta-miokarda.html

[13] Encyclopedia of Cardiology. Available from: http://cardiobook.ru/priznaki-infarkta-miokarda-u-zhenshhin/

[14] Dvoretsky LI, Gibradze NT, Cherkasova NA. Coronary heart disease in women. Russian Medical Journal. 2011;**2**:79-86. https://www.rmj.ru/articles/kardiologiya/Ishemicheskaya_bolezny_serdca_u_ghenschin/#ixzz55l0cbLLG

[15] Boytsov SA, Boytsov S, et al. The Cardiovascular Disease Registry (REKVAZA): Diagnostics, combined cardiovascular pathology, comorbidities, and treatment under real outpatient polyclinic practice. Cardiovascular Therapy and Prevention. 2014;**13**(6):44-50. DOI: 10.15829/1728-8800-2014-6-3-8. ISSN:

2619-0125. Available from: https://cardiovascular.elpub.ru/jour/article/view/81

[16] James MT. Longitudinal studies 4: Matching strategies to evaluate risk. Methods in Molecular Biology. 2015; **1281**:133-143

[17] 5 and 5 Medicine. Triglycerides are elevated, what does this mean? Available from: http://www.5u5.ru/articles/articles-drugs/160-triglitsetidy-kak-faktor-riska.html

[18] Deedwania P, Kosiborod M, Barrett E, et al. Hyperglycemia and acute coronary syndrome: A scientific statement from the American Heart Association Diabetes Committee of the Council on Nutrition, Physical Activity, and Metabolism. Circulation. 2008;**117**: 1610-1619

[19] Abadal AC, Flores JS. The significance of hyperglycemia in acute coronary syndrome. Revista Española de Cardiología. 2008;**61**(5):447-450

[20] Erlich AD, Gratsiansky NA. Independent register of acute coronary syndromes record. Characteristics of patients and treatment before discharge from the hospital. Atherothrombosis. 2009;**1**(2):105-119

[21] Flegal KM, Kit BK, Orpana H, Graubard BI. Association of all-cause mortality with overweight and obesity using standard body mass index categories: A systematic review and meta-analysis. JAMA. 2013;**309**(1):71-82

[22] de Ferranti SD, de Boer IH, Fonseca V, Fox CS, et al. Type 1 diabetes mellitus and cardiovascular disease: A scientific statement from the American Heart Association and American Diabetes Association. Diabetes Care. 2014;**37**(10): 2843-2863

[23] Kotb NA, Gaber R, Salah W, Elhendy A. Relations among glycemic control, circulating endothelial cells, nitric oxide, and flow mediated dilation in patients with type 2 diabetes mellitus. Experimental and Clinical Endocrinology & Diabetes. 2012;**120**(8): 460-465

[24] Podachina SV. From classical therapy of diabetic neuropathy to solving the problem of hyperglycemic memory. Effective pharmacotherapy. Endocrinology. 2012;**1**:48-52

[25] Malmberg K, Rydén L, Efendic S, Herlitz J, Nicol P, Waldenström A, et al. Randomized trial of insulin glucose infusion followed by subcutaneous insulin treatment in diabetic patients with acute myocardial infarction (DIGAMI study): Effects on mortality at 1 year. Journal of the American College of Cardiology. 1995;**26**(1):57-65

[26] Malmberg K, Rydén L, Hamsten A, Herlitz J, Waldenström A, Wedel H. Effects of insulin treatment on cause-specific one year mortality and morbidity in diabetic patients with acute myocardial infarction. DIGAMI Study Group. Diabetes insulin glucose in acute myocardial infarction. European Heart Journal. 1996;**17**(9):1337-1344

[27] Roth GA, Forouzanfar MH, Moran AE, Barber R, Nguyen G, Feigin VL, et al. Demographic and epidemiologic drivers of global cardiovascular mortality. The New England Journal of Medicine. 2015;**372**(14):1333-1341

[28] Wang W, Lau Y, Loo A, et al. Medication adherence and its associated factors among Chinese community-dwelling older adults with hypertension. Heart & Lung. 2014;**43**(4):278-283

[29] Fodor GJ, Kotrec M, Bacskai K, et al. Is interview a reliable method to verify the compliance with antihypertensive therapy? An international Central-European study. Journal of Hypertension. 2005;**23**:1261-1266

[30] Rao CR, Veena KG, Shetty A, et al. Treatment compliance among patients with hypertension and type 2 diabetes mellitus in a coastal population of Southern India. International Journal of Preventive Medicine. 2014;**5**(8):992-998

[31] Raymundo NAC, Pierin AMG. Adherence to anti-hypertensive treatment within a chronic disease management program: A longitudinal, retrospective study. Revista da Escola de Enfermagem da U.S.P. 2014;**48**(5): 809-881

Chapter 5

Ontology-Based Modeling for Newborn Behavior Simulation during Cardiopulmonary Resuscitation

Jean-Marc Mercantini

Abstract

This chapter concerns the formulation of a methodology and its implementation to elaborate a training simulator for medical staff who may be confronted with the critical situations of newborn resuscitation. The simulator reproduces the different cardiopulmonary pathological behaviors of newborns, the working environment of resuscitation rooms, and the monitoring and control environment of the learners by a teacher. Conceptual models of newborn behaviors combined with the cardiopulmonary resuscitation gestures have been developed. The methodological process is jointly using cognitive approaches with formal modeling and simulation. Cognitive approaches are mobilized to elaborate application ontologies to be the bases for the development of the conceptual models and the specification of the simulator. Ontologies have been developed on the bases of a corpus of academic documents, return on experience documents, and practitioner interviews, by means of the knowledge-oriented design (KOD) method. A discrete event formalism has been used to formalize the conceptual models of the newborn behaviors. As a result, a simulator has been built to train medical practitioners to face situations, which are reported to potentially cause errors, and thus improve the safety of the resuscitation gestures.

Keywords: newborn resuscitation, clinician training, ontology engineering, conceptual modeling, discrete event modeling, simulation

1. Introduction

Approximately 15% of newborns require respiratory support at birth, and 2% require complex resuscitation (intubation, chest compression, and/or epinephrine) [1]. In France, 25% of the causes of neonatal mortality are due to respiratory difficulties: intrauterine hypoxia, asphyxia at birth, respiratory distress syndrome, or other respiratory diseases.

Given these emergencies at birth, specialized technical equipment and skilled personnel are required to carry out all or part of the following procedures [1]: (i) the initial stage of stabilization (airway clearance, neonatal placement, and stimulation), (ii) ventilation, (iii) chest compressions, and (iv) medication or volume expansion.

These procedures are well known and quite simple to implement and execute. Criticality of induced situations is due to time constraints, stress, and the fact that they are not frequent situations. Medical personnel have to analyze the situation, diagnose the problem, and perform the "right" actions within 60 seconds after birth to avoid critical delays in initiation of resuscitation [1]. A diagnostic or execution error can lead to irreversible damage or death. The problem is that despite the rarity of these situations, they require highly trained medical personnel.

The "Cyber-Poupon" project, from the Ab Initio Medical company, is an answer to this problem of personnel qualification. It consists in designing and developing an integrated simulation system for the training of medical staff who may be confronted with the critical situations of resuscitation of newborns.

Currently, the main instrumented anatomical simulators of newborns are marketed by the companies Laerdal, Simulaids, CAE, Gaumard, or Medical-X. They all contain a large number of configurable physiological functions and most pathological behavioral scenarios of the newborn. These simulators are now widely used in resuscitation training centers. However, there are still many gaps that can interfere with learning objectives:

- Lack of realism in physical appearance (materials and resemblance)
- Lack of realism of the dynamic aspect (behavior, movements, and reactivity)
- Nonautomatic evaluation of the learner's gestures (reaction of the robot to resuscitation actions)

These inadequacies necessarily induce learner's behaviors too far from what they must master in real situations. These shortcomings have led the responsible staff in charge of the neonatology service, from the "Conception" Hospital in Marseilles, to develop their own simulation system jointly with the Ab Initio Medical company, and in partnership with the "Data Processing and Systems Laboratory" (Laboratoire d'Informatique et Systèmes (LIS)) from Aix-Marseille University.

The current work lies in the following research fields: (1) from the medical field perspective, the paper presents a software tool (simulator) to train medical staff to cardiopulmonary resuscitation gestures to improve newborn safety and (2) from a methodological perspective, the paper shows the importance of developing ontologies (i) for structuring a domain (at a conceptual level) as its actors perceive it and (ii) for using these ontologies to build computer tools with pedagogical perspective in that domain.

An overview of the newborn resuscitation is presented in Section 2, and Section 3 presents the Cyber-Poupon project. Section 4 describes the methodological approach and the process used to build the simulator. In Section 5, the implementation of the process is developed and exemplified. Section 6 presents the conclusions.

2. The newborn resuscitation

2.1 Situations giving rise to resuscitation

The transition from fetal life to extrauterine life is characterized by a series of events: the lungs move from an aquatic environment to an air environment, pulmonary blood flow increases significantly and shunts through the oval foramen, and the arterial canal changes direction and then closes. This complex process may be hampered by (i) a failure of normalization of the pulmonary vascular resistance, (ii) a lack of alveolar opening, and (iii) a premature birth and may provoke respiratory distress at birth requiring resuscitation.

Beyond these functional impediments, many other situations can lead to resuscitation in the workplace: maternal situations (such as drug addiction, diabetes, hypertension, chronic diseases, etc.), fetal situations (such as prematurity, post-maturity, intravenous infection, etc.), and obstetric situations (such as prolonged work, fast work, forceps delivery, cesarean delivery, etc.). In addition to birth cases identified as potentially requiring resuscitation, all births require the presence of at least one person trained to perform initial care and who will only take care of one newborn. She must be able to start resuscitation, including positive pressure ventilation and chest compressions.

2.2 The neonatal evaluation-resuscitation process

The International Liaison Committee on Resuscitation (ILCOR) publishes regularly recommendations on the management of newborns at birth [1]. Among these recommendations a newborn assessment-resuscitation process is provided (**Figure 1**), highlighting the questions that practitioners need to ask themselves, as well as resuscitation techniques to be undertaken. If the newborn does not require resuscitation (case 1), only routine care will be provided. If not (case 2), the newborn will probably need to receive one or more of the following actions [1]:

A. Initial steps in stabilization (clearing the airway, positioning, stimulating)

B. Ventilation

C. Chest compressions

D. Medication or volume expansion

During this process, the practitioner observes the vital functions: breathing, heart rate, color (which results from the two previous ones), and tone. The steps of resuscitation follow one another stereotypically in the same order: (1) clear the airways by aspiration, head posture, stimulations; (2) ventilation; (3) chest compressions; (4) and adrenaline and/or volume expansion. Each step lasts approximately 30 seconds. **Figure 1** shows a flowchart form of this evaluation-resuscitation process.

2.3 Overview of the resuscitation technics

Clearing airway: it consists in positioning the newborn on the back and tilting the head slightly backwards by raising the chin. This gesture can be complemented (if necessary) by secretion suctioning.

Ventilation: it consists in increasing the air or oxygen supply of the newborn. It aims to increase alveolar ventilation, improve gas exchange, and reduce the work of the respiratory muscles. Diverse ventilation techniques are available:

- The oxygen supplementation
- Nasal ventilation (positive pressure and noninvasive)
- Manual ventilation with mask (positive pressure and noninvasive)
- Manual ventilation on intubation probe (positive pressure and invasive)
- Mechanized ventilation on intubation probe (positive pressure and invasive)

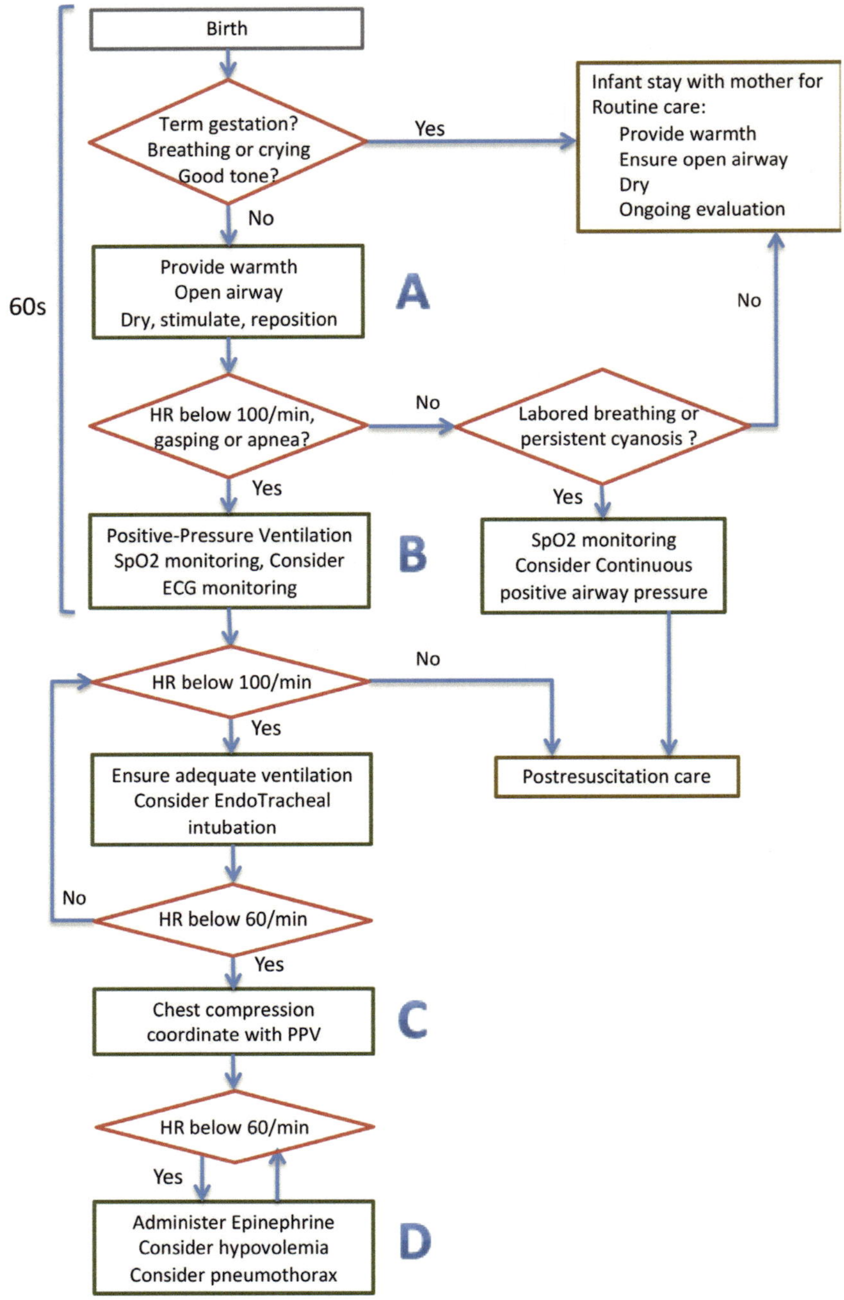

Figure 1.
ILCOR neonatal flow algorithm from [1, 2] where red triangles are evaluation actions and green boxes are resuscitation actions.

Nasotracheal intubation: it consists in introducing a probe (or cannula) through the mouth (or nose) of the newborn until it penetrates the trachea. A ventilation system can then be connected directly to the probe.

Chest compression: it consists in rhythmic compressions of the sternum that compresses the heart against the spine. It aims to ensure a blood flow from the heart to the vital organs. The compressions should be made on the lower third of the sternum, and the thorax should be sink up to a depth of about 2 cm. Ventilation should be continued during chest compression.

Medication: it is rarely indicated during newborn resuscitation. In some cases (low heart rate despite good ventilation), it may be appropriate to administer epinephrine (adrenaline) or to proceed to a volume expansion.

3. The Cyber-Poupon project

The “Cyber-Poupon” project consists in developing a realistic simulation system designed to train hospital agents to the resuscitation gestures of newborns suffering from cardiopulmonary pathologies. The simulation system reproduces the different pathological behaviors of a newborn (newborn simulator), the working environment of a resuscitation room (resuscitation environment simulator), and the monitoring and control environment of the learner by a teacher (monitoring and control system) (**Figure 2**).

Two categories of exercises are possible: (i) targeted training on one or more specific gestures (intubation, ventilation, etc.) and (ii) training in the diagnosis of a pathology followed by planning a protocol and its execution.

In the first class of exercises, the professor chooses the gesture(s) to be executed (see (1) in **Figure 2**), and in the second class of exercises, the professor chooses a scenario corresponding to a pathology (1). In both cases, the simulator generates the gesture reference model (2) and the Cyber-Poupon behavior model (3) automatically. The comparison between the reference model of the gestures to be realized and the way they are actually performed produces a gap whose sign and amplitude will induce a new state of the Cyber-Poupon. This state is returned to the learner by visualizing physiological variables such as oxygen saturation (SPO2) or heart rate (4). The learner then adjusts his gestures (5) according to his analysis of this feedback. The teacher, through his monitoring and control system, receives the same information as the learner and can act directly on the learner’s monitoring system (6). A set of cameras records the learner’s work as the basis for the debriefing following the simulation session.

The simulation system belongs to the category of “instrumented anatomical simulator” in reference to the classification of medical simulators proposed by [3]:

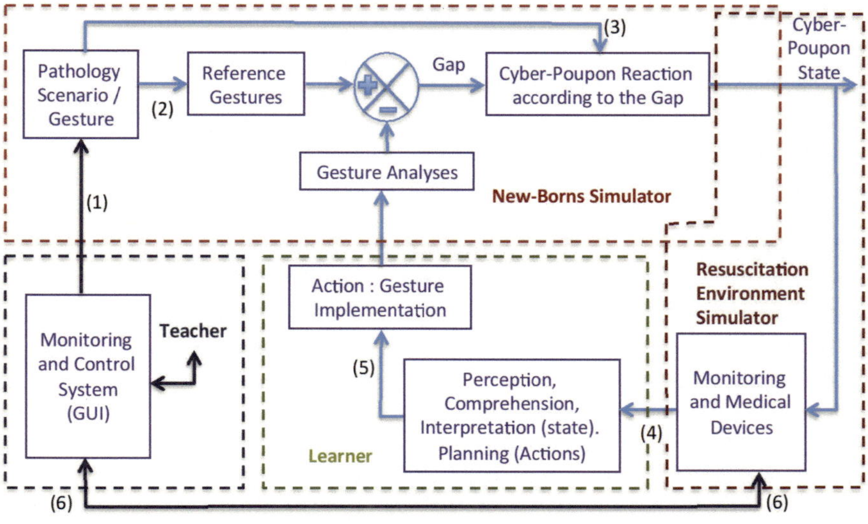

Figure 2.
Functional diagram of the newborn simulation system. Relationships labeled with a number between brackets (n) are detailed in the above paragraph.

- Virtual simulators with a 3D graphical user interface (3D GUI)
- Virtual simulators with a 3D GUI and coupled to a force feedback system
- Anatomical simulators consisting of a non-instrumented dummy
- Instrumented anatomical simulators (IAS)

IAS simulators consist of an instrumented dummy ("newborn simulator"—**Figure 2**) and can be supplemented by a virtual interface ("resuscitation environment simulator" and "monitoring and control system"—**Figure 2**). They are recognized to provide a more realistic immersion of the learners.

Simulated reactions of the Cyber-Poupon are in accordance with the following learner's gestures: (1) manual ventilation with mask (bag-mask ventilation), (2) nasal ventilation, (3) manual ventilation on intubation probe, (4) mechanized ventilation on intubation probe, (5) nasotracheal intubation, (6) tracheal suctioning, (7) nasopharyngeal clearance, (8) gastric emptying, (9) extubation, (10) and chest compressions.

4. Methodological approach

4.1 Analysis of the problem

Conception of new computer tools with pedagogical objectives requires deep reflexions about transmission and content. A wrong way to transmit or a wrong system of concepts (wrong content) can lead to "dormant fault" in the learner's cognitive system, which will be activated during work situations. For newborn resuscitation activities, it could lead to fatal accidents. The notion of ontology and works currently developed by the knowledge engineers community can bring interesting answers to this problem [4, 5].

First defined in metaphysics, ontology studies being or existence and their basic categories and relationships, to determine what entities and what types of entities exist [6]. In formalizing the nature of things and the distinctions between them, ontology is applied to fields such as theology, information science, and artificial intelligence [7]. The ontology field studies the world as an organization of its fundamental categories and their interrelationships [8].

Within computer science domain, ontology is often associated to knowledge related to objects of a delimited universe and their relations. Ontology refers to a conceptual language used for the description of this delimited universe (domain). The emergence of this notion in knowledge-based system (KBS) engineering comes from the fact that the way to observe the world and its interpretation depend on the observer culture, his (her) means to observe it as well as to his (her) intentions. In this sense, it becomes necessary to resolve the difficulties caused by observation, representation, and interpretation of (normal or critic) situations to facilitate problem solving (intent).

Definitions given by Gruber and Ushold are very pertinent in the context of pedagogical objectives: (1) "an ontology is an explicit specification of a conceptualization, defined as an abstract simplified view of the world that one wishes to represent for some purpose" [8, 9], and (2) "One of the objectives of ontologies is to facilitate the exchange of knowledge between humans, between humans and machines as well as humans via machines" [10].

General benefits in developing ontologies for solving problems arising in the field of safety and Health care are the following:

- They structure the domain in highlighting concepts and semantic relations that are linking these concepts.
- They can be used to be the base for new computer tool design.
- They can be used to be the base for new pedagogical approaches.

More specific benefits (linked to the application) can be highlighted, such as:

- Deep and guided analysis and modeling of the diverse pathological scenario
- Deep and guided analysis and modeling of the diverse protocols (gestures, instruments, and reasoning)
- Deep and guided analysis and modeling of the newborn behaviors
- Deep and guided analysis of the pedagogical tools to implement
- Setting out and modeling the reference gestures and protocols

Tools so built are carrying knowledge shared by the actors of the domain (professionals, professors, and learners), which makes them more effective to train medical staff to the right gestures within critical situations. The discourse is not to say that it is not possible to properly conceive new intelligent systems without using ontologies, but the use of ontologies obliges designers to follow a deep and guided methodological analysis of the problems to be solved and to express them by means of the right system of concepts.

Ontologies can also be defined according to their level of genericity as proposed by Guarino in [11]. The so-called top-level ontologies describe very generic concepts independent of any particular problem or domain. They must be "reusable from one domain to another and are designed to reduce inconsistencies in terms defined downstream" [12]. Domain ontologies and task ontologies, respectively, describe the concepts of a generic domain (such as medicine, industrial production, etc.) or the concepts of a generic task or problem (such as diagnosis, prognosis, planning, simulation, etc.). They specialize terms introduced by top-level ontologies.

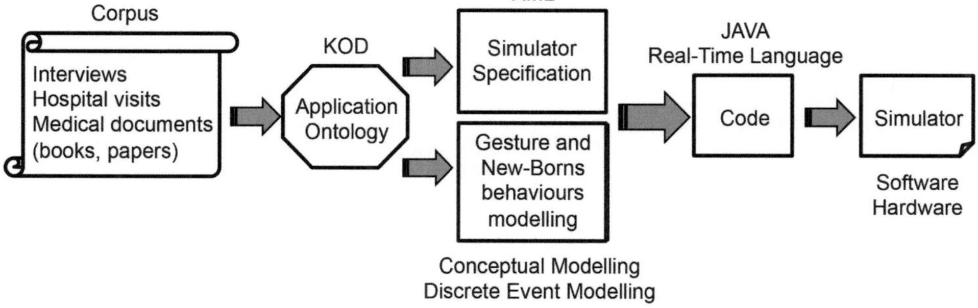

Figure 3.
The implemented methodological process.

Application ontologies (the most specific) describe concepts related to a task (or problem) occurring in a particular domain (such as medical diagnosis or planning). They are both a union and a specialization of ontologies of tasks and domains.

The proposed methodological process (**Figure 3**) consists in adopting approaches and methods from knowledge engineering (KE) combined with formal modeling. It consists in developing application ontology aiming to model in a unified way the triplet Td: <Domain, Problem, Method>. In this sense, the ontology structures the domain according to the problem to be solved and taking into account the problem solving methods. The application ontology is the foundation for the development of the conceptual models of the newborn resuscitation (medical gesture and newborn behaviors) and the specification of the simulator. The process is based on the "knowledge-oriented design" (KOD) method [13, 14].

4.2 The KOD method

KOD was designed to introduce an explicit conceptual model (the cognitive model) between the formulation of a software tool expressed in natural language and its representation in a formal language (the software model). The inductive process of KOD is based on the analysis of a corpus of documents, comments, and experts' statements, describing the different aspects of the problem to solve (raw data). The fundamental bases of this method are coming from linguistics and cognitive anthropology. Its linguistic bases make it well suited for the acquisition of knowledge expressed in natural language. For this, KOD proposes a methodological framework to guide the acquisition of pertinent terms from the corpus and to organize them by means of a terminological analysis (linguistic capacity). Thanks to its anthropological bases, KOD provides a methodological framework to guide the semantic analysis of the terminology to produce a cognitive model (conceptualization capacity). KOD guides work from knowledge extraction up to the software model via the cognitive model development.

The implementing process of KOD requires the development of three kinds of successive models: the practical models, the cognitive model, and the software model (**Table 1**). Each one is developed according to the three paradigms: representation, action, and interpretation/intention.

The representation paradigm provides KOD with the ability to model the knowledge of the domain such perceived and interiorized by actors. This knowledge universe is made of concrete or abstract objects in relation. KOD provides methodological tools to develop the structure of this universe according to this paradigm. The action paradigm provides KOD with the ability to model the behavior of active objects that activate procedures upon receipt of messages. Action plans designed and performed by human actors, as well as those performed by artificial actors, are

Paradigms models	Representation	Action	Interpretation
Practical	Taxeme: object static representation	Acteme: dynamic representation of active objects	Inferences
Cognitive	Taxonomy: object static organization according to their properties	Actinomy: dynamic object organization	Reasoning pattern
Software	Classes	Methods	Rules

Table 1.
The KOD modeling space.

modeled with the same format. The interpretation/intention paradigm provides KOD with the ability to model the reasoning patterns used by human or artificial actors to interpret situations and elaborate action plans related to their intentions (reasoning capacity).

Practical models are the representation of a speech or document expressed in the terms of the domain, by means of "taxemes" (static representation of objects—French word), "actemes" (dynamic representation of objects—French word), and inferences (basic element of the cognitive reasoning pattern). A "taxeme" is a minimum grammatical feature; it is the verbalization of an object or a class of objects. An "acteme" is the verbalization of an act or a transformation, a unit of behavior. An inference is the act or process of deriving logical conclusions from premises known or assumed to be true. The cognitive model is an abstraction of the practical models. It is composed of taxonomies, actinomies, and reasoning patterns. The software model results from the formalization of the cognitive model expressed in a formal language independently of any programming language.

4.3 Elaboration of the models

The first step consists in developing practical models (Mp_i). Based on a corpus of documents (D_i) (**Figure 4**), it consists in extracting terms and relations linking them through a terminological analysis to provide a terminological language. The terms of this language are classified into taxemes, actemes, and inferences consistent with the three paradigms of the method (**Table 1**). At the end of this first step of the modeling process, each document of the corpus (D_1, D_2, ..., D_n) is modeled by means of a practical model (MP_1, MP_2, ..., MP_n) (**Figure 4**). Each practical model is a representation of a specific case or aspect or point of view of the problem such perceived or lived by actors of the domain.

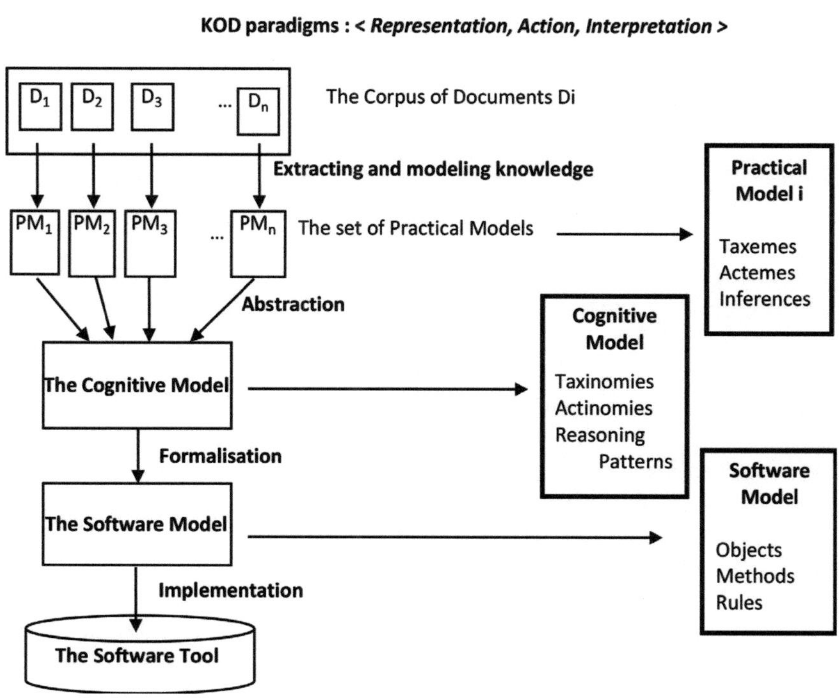

Figure 4.
The KOD design process.

The second step consists in developing the cognitive model related to the problem, from the set of practical models. The process consists in (i) analyzing synonyms and homonyms terms occurring in the practical models, (ii) determining the pertinent identifier terms, (iii) transforming the resulting terms into concepts, and (iv) transforming the lexical relationships into semantic ones. In accordance with the three paradigms of the method, the cognitive model is made of taxonomies, actinomies, and reasoning patterns (**Figure 4**). Taxonomies result from taxeme classification as a hierarchical tree structure showing connections between concepts and objects. Actinomies result from an orderly organization of actemes defining an action plan. Reasoning patterns are modeling human reasoning leading to action planning before executing them. The KOD process encourages the emergence of generic and consensual characteristics of the conceptual language with which the cognitive model is expressed. Indeed, solving synonymy and homonymy problems promotes consensual characteristics, and abstractions of practical models promote obtaining a conceptual and generic language.

The third step concerns the development of the software model requiring to previously translate the cognitive model by means of a formal language. The choice of the formal language depends on the properties of the conceptual model and of the methods implemented by the software tool to solve the problem. The formalization operation consists in integrating the elements of the conceptual model in the definition of classes and objects to constitute the formal model to be used for the software development. The implementation phase that follows consists in translating the formal model by means of a programming language.

4.4 The ontology building process using KOD

Research work in ontology engineering has put in evidence five main steps for building ontologies [10, 15–18]:

1. *Ontology specification*. It consists in providing a description of the problem as well as the method to solve it. Objectives, scope, and granularity of the ontology to be developed are discussed and specified.

2. *Corpus definition*. It consists in selecting information sources, which will allow the objectives of the study to be reached.

3. *Linguistic study of the corpus*. It consists in a terminological analysis to extract relevant terms and their relations. Linguistics is especially concerned to the extent that available data for ontology building are often expressed in natural language. Characterization of the sense of these linguistic expressions leads to determine contextual meanings.

4. *Conceptualization*. Relevant terms and their relations resulting from the linguistic study are analyzed. Terms are transformed into concepts, and their lexical relations are transformed into semantic relations. The result is a conceptual model.

5. *Formalization*. It consists in expressing the conceptual model by means of a formal language.

Projection of the KOD method on the general approach of ontology development shows that KOD guides the constitution of the corpus and provides tools

Elaboration process of ontology	KOD process	Elaboration process of ontology with KOD
1. Specification 2. Corpus definition 3. Linguistic study 4. Conceptualization 5. Formalization	1. Practical model 2. Cognitive model 3. Software model	1. Specification 2. Corpus definition 3. Practical model 4. Cognitive model 5. Formalization 6. Software model

Table 2.
Integration of the KOD method into the elaboration process of ontology.

to answer the operational stages 3 (linguistic study) and 4 (conceptualization) (**Table 2**). To illustrate ontology building using KOD, the following previous works can be cited: aircraft piloting errors [19], accidental seaside pollution [20], or simulation of supply chain vulnerability [21].

5. Elaboration of the ontology for the Cyber-Poupon

5.1 Ontology specification

The KOD method does not offer tools facilitating the specification of ontology. To carry out this step, many authors recommend the use of the scenario concept [10, 18, 22] with the objectives to clarify and justify the ontology development, its future uses, and its future addressees. This step will not be further developed, but it is illustrated by giving summaries of the scenario that have been drafted within the framework of the triplet Td: <Domain, Problem, Method>.

The domain is that of newborn cardiopulmonary resuscitation. The problem is to train medical staff to produce the right diagnosis, the right gesture planning, and execution. The problem solving method consists in the elaboration of a cooperative system of simulation. The ontology has to structure the domain with regard to the problem to be solved and taking into account the problem solving method. The ontology realizes the coherence of the triplet Td to serve as a basis for the design of the simulation tool. In this sense, it is important that the elaborating method of the ontology helps to conceptualize the triplet Td.

5.2 Corpus definition

Definition and analysis of the corpus are based on the ontology specification and on the properties of the practical and cognitive models resulting from the application of the KOD method. Thus, documents to be collected must be both representative of the triplet: <Domain, Problem, Method> and meet the requirements induced by the KOD modeling space (**Table 1**). The combination of the triplet (Td) with the KOD modeling space constitutes a helpful grid to analyze the ontology specification with the goal to define the documents of the corpus. The corpus is made of the following documents:

- Professional documents about medical protocols
- Academic documents about the resuscitation gestures
- Technical documents about the main instrumented anatomical simulators of newborns

- Interviews concerning the return on operating experience about well-done resuscitation
- Interviews concerning the return on operating experience about erroneously done resuscitation

5.3 Elaboration of the practical models

This step consists in extracting, from each document of the corpus, relevant knowledge (objects, actions, and inferences) for modeling newborn pathological behaviors combined with the cardiopulmonary resuscitation gestures.

5.3.1 Taxemes modeling

The linguistic analysis is performed in two steps: verbalization and modeling into taxemes. Verbalization consists in paraphrasing corpus documents in order to obtain simple sentences allowing to qualify the employed terms. Terms are referring to objects, concepts, properties, values, or relationships between objects and values. Modeling consists in organizing paraphrases by means of binary predicates such as object, attribute, and value, where attribute defines a relationship between the object and a value.

Five kinds of predicative relationships are defined: classifying (is-a, kind-of), identifying (is), descriptive (position, failure mode, error mode, cause, etc.), structural (composed-of), and situational (is-in, is-below, etc.). The following example illustrates the process to obtain the taxemes in the case of the "Bag-Mask Ventilation" gesture. The extract is translated from [23]:

"Two types of manual insufflators are presented: AMBU type and Leardal type. Their design, principles and uses are roughly similar."

"...They are made of: the balloon, the injection and exhalation valves, the pressure relief valve, the universal patient connector, and the oxygen connection. ...".

Paraphrases:

1. The "AMBU manual insufflator" is a manual insufflator.
2. The "Leardal manual insufflator" is a manual insufflator.
3. "Manual insufflator" is made of a balloon.
4. "Manual insufflator" is made of an injection valve.
5. "Manual insufflator" is made of an exhalation valve.
6. etc.

Taxemes:

1. <AMBU manual insufflator, *kind-of*, Manual insufflator>
2. < Leardal manual insufflator, *kind-of*, Manual insufflator >
3. < Manual insufflator, *composed-of*, Balloon>
4. < Manual insufflator, *composed-of*, Injection valve >

5. < Manual insufflator, *composed-of*, Exhalation valve >

6. etc.

Two predicative relationships are used in this extract: the classifying and structural relationships. The extent of this analysis at the whole corpus has allowed obtaining the set of taxemes needed for the representation of the newborn resuscitation universe. Each object of the real world is modeled by the set of the related taxemes (**Figure 5**).

5.3.2 Acteme modeling

Actemes are modeling resuscitation activities, as well as newborn and object behaviors. In order to obtain actemes, the linguistic analysis consists in identifying verbs that represent activities performed by the medical staff during resuscitation, newborn behaviors or object behaviors. An activity is performed by an action manager, by means of instruments, to modify the state (physical or knowledge) of the addressee. An acteme is composed of textual items extracted from the corpus, which describe the state changing of an entity as described by domain experts. The following example illustrates how to extract actemes from the corpus:

"... The manual bag mask ventilation is carried out by means of a manual insufflator by exerting repeated compressions of the balloon (50 cycles per minute for the new-born and 30 cycles per minute for the infant ..."

The activity (or action) is "Manual Bag-Mask Ventilation." Once identified, the activity is translated into a 7-tuple (the acteme). Each element of the 7-tuple must be previously defined as a taxeme:

<Action Name, Action Manager, Addressee, Properties, State 1, State 2, Instruments>

where

- Action Manager (clinician or learner) performs the action (Action Name).
- Action (action name) causes the change.
- Addressee (newborn or Cyber-Poupon) undergoes the action.

Extract of the New-Born taxemes

<New-Born, *Composed-of*, Limbs>
<New-Born, *Composed-of*, Face>
...
<New-Born, *Composed-of*, Epiglottis>
<New-Born, *Composed-of*, Trachea>
...
<New-Born, *Composed-of*, Lungs>

Physiological components of the new-born implied in respiratory failure and resuscitation (Structural relation)

...
<New-Born, *OxygenSaturation*, Real_Value>
<New-Born, *HeartRate*, Real_Value>
<New-Born, *RespiratoryFrequence*, Real_Value>
<New-Born, *BloodPressure*, Real_Value>
<New-Born, *Colour*, Set_of_Colours>
<New-Born, *Tonicity*, Discretised_Levels>
...

Physiological variables of the new-born implied in respiratory failure and resuscitation (Descriptive relation)

Figure 5.
A subset of the newborn taxemes.

- Properties describe the way the action is performed.
- State 1 is the state of the addressee before the change.
- State 2 is the state of the addressee after the change.
- Instruments are used to cause the change (the insufflator).

The acteme "Manual Bag-Mask Ventilation" is represented as follows:

<Manual Bag-Mask Ventilation, Learner, Cyber-Poupon, (Cycles, Regularity, Duration, Volume, MaxPressure), Cyber-Poupon (Not Ventilated), Cyber-Poupon (Ventilated), AMBU Manual Insufflator>

Actemes can be represented according to an actigram form (**Figure 6**) or to a table form (**Table 3**).

The Cyber-Poupon state, summarized in **Figure 6** by the terms "Not Ventilated" and "Ventilated", is in fact a subset of the Cyber-Poupon attributes (the physiological variables) that are affected by a respiratory failure and consequently, by a bag-mask ventilation. The action manager evaluates the physiological state of the Cyber-Poupon, through the analysis of the following vector:

(Oxygen Saturation, Heart rate, Respiratory Frequency, Blood pressure, Color, Tonicity, Screams)

Values taken by each attribute (physiological variables) evolve according to the right or wrong realization of the considered resuscitation gesture (action): the "Manual Bag-Mask Ventilation" in the case of the example. Properties of the action characterize the way the action is performed (**Figure 10**), where

- Cycles is the gesture frequency (number of cycles per minute).
- Regularity is the constant of the performed gestures.

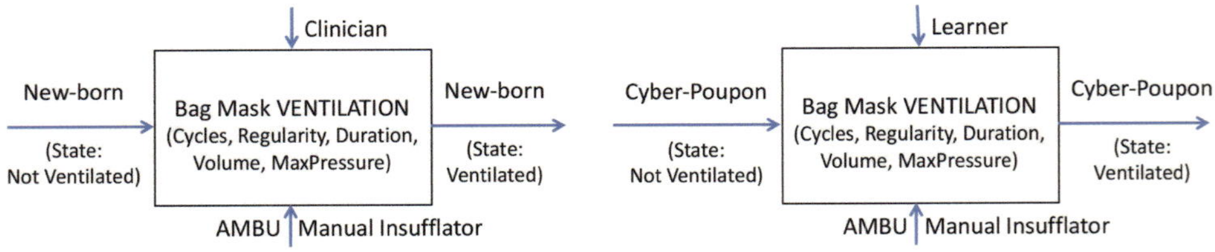

Figure 6.
Representation of the acteme "Manual Bag-Mask Ventilation" according to an actigram form. Modeling in real situation on the left-hand side and modeling in learning situation on the right-hand side.

Action: Manual Bag-Mask Ventilation	
Components	**Values**
Action Manager	{Learner, Professor, Clinician}
Addressee	{Cyber-Poupon, Newborn}
Addressee State 1	{Not Ventilated}
Addressee State 2	{Ventilated}
Instruments	{AMBU Manual Insufflator, Leardal Manual Insufflator}
Properties	{Cycles, Regularity, Duration, Volume, MaxPressure}

Table 3.
Representation of the acteme "Manual Bag-Mask Ventilation" according to a table form.

- Duration is the elapsed time during the balloon compression.
- Volume is the quantity of air or oxygen insufflated in lungs.
- MaxPressure is the maximal pressure exercised by the clinician (or learner) during the manual compression of the balloon.

The evaluation of these properties gives a measure of the right or wrong realization of the "Manual Bag-Mask Ventilation" gesture.

5.4 The cognitive model (conceptualization)

Conceptualization consists in developing the cognitive model by abstraction of the practical models. It is based on the operation of classification to produce taxonomies, actinomies, and reasoning patterns.

5.4.1 Taxonomy building

The first step consists in solving problems induced by homonym and synonym terms, with the objective to build a coherent and common terminology. The second step consists in analyzing the nature of attributes (or relationships) that characterize each object. From the nature of these attributes, the building of taxonomies (relationships "kind-of" or "is-a") or other kinds of tree structures (relationships "is-composed-of", "is-on", etc.) will depend.

According to the previous example, the following can be initiated: (1) the manual insufflator taxonomy where AMBU manual insufflator and Leardal manual insufflator are *kind-of* manual insufflators and (2) a tree structure giving the composition of a manual insufflator (**Figure 7**), which is included in a wider tree structure (ventilation system). All taxemes of the corpus have been organized in taxonomies and tree structures to express all the relationships between concepts.

The definition of a concept is achieved by combining the whole knowledge about it. As a result of the analysis of the knowledge related to "AMBU manual insufflator," the concept is defined through its attributes as shown in **Table 4**.

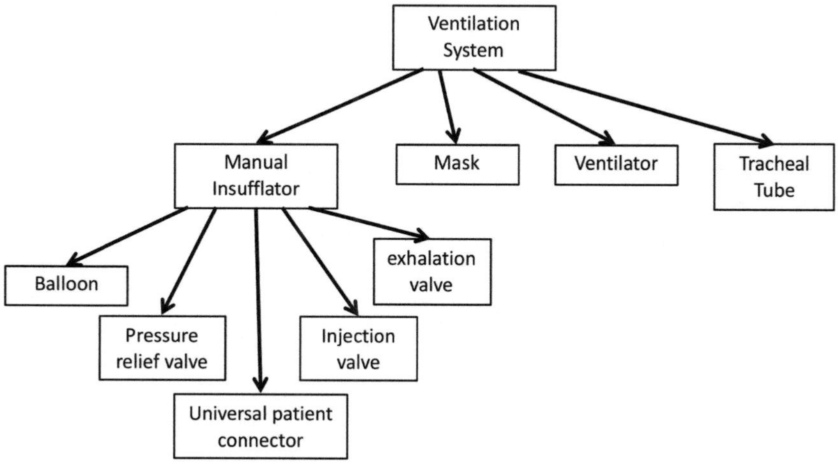

Figure 7.
Tree structure based on the "composed-of" relation.

Manual insufflator	
Attributes	**Values**
Kind-of	Manual insufflator
Composed-of	Balloon
Composed-of	Pressure valve
Composed-of	Universal patient connector
Composed-of	Injection valve
Composed-of	Exhalation valve
Balloon volume	Real
Balloon compliance	Real
Gas nature	{Oxygen, air}

Table 4.
The attributes of the "manual insufflator" concept.

5.4.2 Acteme abstraction

One result of the acteme analysis is that they can be classified into three main action categories: (i) actions related to newborn behaviors, (ii) actions related to resuscitation gestures, and (iii) actions related to pedagogical services.

Actions related to newborn behaviors are executed by the Cyber-Poupon as a result of the physiological state changes induced by the learner resuscitation gestures. Such actions include tonicity change, heart rate change, SPO2 change, etc.

Actions related to resuscitation gestures are executed by the clinician, and they have to be captured and qualified by the Cyber-Poupon. Each of these actions has been deeply analyzed to elaborate the qualification process. Examples of such actions include manual bag-mask ventilation, nasotracheal intubation, tracheal aspiration, gastric emptying, chest compression, etc.

The actions related to pedagogical services are implemented to improve the simulator functionalities to assist the professor in its supervising and debriefing tasks such as recording a simulation session, inserting comments during a simulation session, etc.

The acteme abstraction has led to two kinds of organization: action taxonomies and actinomies. As an example, **Figure 8** presents the taxonomy of the ventilation actions. Some actemes of the resuscitation gesture can be organized in a structural and temporal way to form actinomies. The interest of this kind of structure is that a set of actions is already planned and they can be used as reference models (**Figure 9**) for a whole process. Thanks to the modeling facilities offered by actemes and actinomies, the development process of the gesture reference models (**Figure 1**, label (2)) has been made simplified. The gesture reference models are so composed of individual actemes as reference models of atomic resuscitation actions and actinomies as reference models of a whole process (**Figure 9**).

5.4.3 Building of reasoning patterns

Reasoning patterns are made of logical inferences to form a coherent complex reasoning. Inferences are modeling knowledge elements of the corpus that characterize cognitive activities of humans and machines. They are the basic elements of the interpretation/intention paradigm.

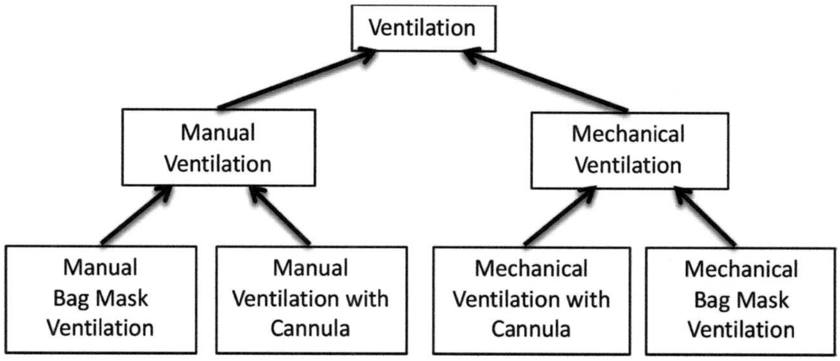

Figure 8.
Extract of the resuscitation gestures taxonomy centered on the ventilation gesture ("kind-of" relation).

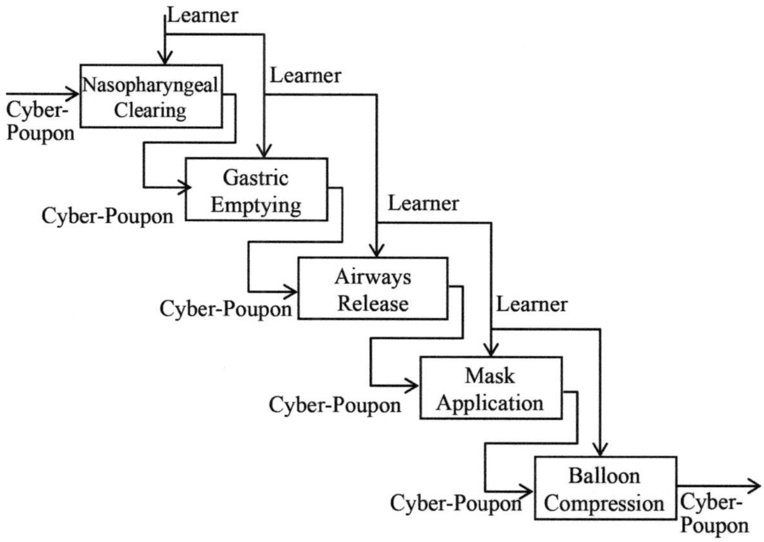

Figure 9.
Simplified representation of the "Manual Bag-Mask Ventilation" actinomy.

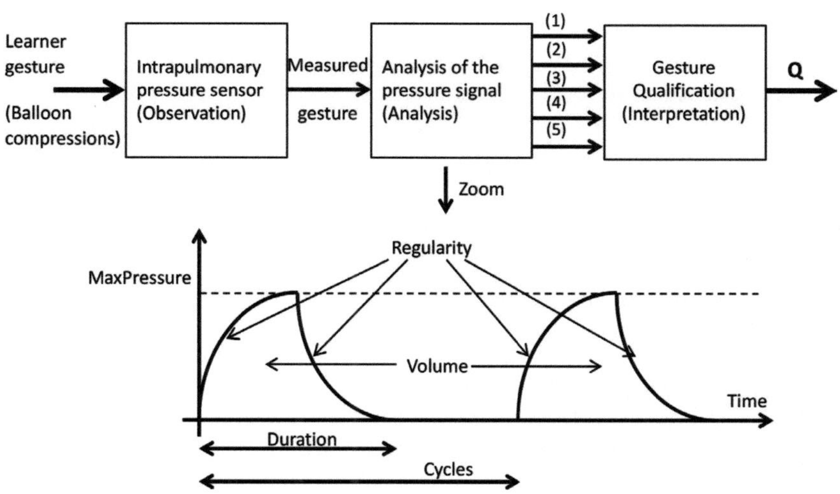

Figure 10.
Qualification of the learner gesture (observation, analysis, interpretation). (n) are the gesture properties: (1) cycles, (2) regularity, (3) duration, (4) volume, (5) MaxPressure. Q is the qualification variable.

To illustrate this step of the methodological process, an extract of the newborn behavioral analysis has been chosen. The example is focused on the "balloon compression" action within the "Manual Bag-Mask Ventilation" (**Figure 10**). As a result, a set of inferences (reasoning pattern) has been stated to control the Cyber-Poupon behaviors in response to the learner gestures. Inferences are built according to the "interpretation/intention" paradigm of the KOD method, and they are expressed according to the following general form:

IF (Interpretation) THEN (Intention)
IF (Interpretation of the Learner gesture(s)) THEN (Generate the induced Cyber-Poupon behavior(s))

The interpretation paradigm addresses observations of the learner gesture(s), and the intention paradigm consists in planning "pseudo-physiological" discrete states with the corresponding behavior(s). Premise propositions result from the interpretation of observations (learner gestures), and therefore, they are held to be true. The conclusion is related to "pseudo-physiological" state transitions.

Figure 10 highlights the Interpretation process where the gesture qualification is based on the gesture properties analysis. The Q variable is the result of the interpretation process, and values taken are [1, 0, −1], where

- $Q = Q_1 = 1$ means that the gesture is rightly executed (positive value).
- $Q = Q_0 = 0$ means no gesture is executed (null value).
- $Q = Q_{-1} = -1$ means that the gesture is wrongly executed (negative value).

For each state of the Cyber-Poupon, the following rules are describing the state transition function:

IF (Q_1 and x_i and elapsetime = dt_{1i}) THEN e_1; (Improvement)
IF (Q_0 and x_i and elapsetime = dt_{0i}) THEN e_0; (Degradation)
IF (Q_{-1} and x_i and elapsetime = dt_{-1i}) THEN e_{-1}; (Degradation)
IF (elapsetime = dt_{inti}) THEN e_{inti}; (Degradation)

where x_i is the current state of the Cyber-Poupon, elapsetime is the time function, dt_{1i} is the necessary right execution duration of the gesture to produce an improvement transition (e_1), dt_{0i} is the duration after which no gesture produce a degradation transition (e_0), dt_{-1i} is the duration after which a wrong execution of the gesture produce a degradation transition (e_{-1}), and dt_{inti} is the time spent in the state i without enough improvement of the physiological variables.

For each state of the Cyber-Poupon, the output functions, which describe the newborn behavior, depend on the right or wrong execution of the gesture. The rules for the output functions are the following:

IF Q_1 and x_i THEN λ_{1i}
IF Q_0 and x_i THEN λ_{0i}
IF Q_{-1} and x_i THEN λ_{-1i}

where λ_{1i}, λ_{0i}, and λ_{-1i} are the sets of output functions associated to the state x_i according to Q_1, Q_0, and Q_{-1}. These functions are modeling the physiological variables of a newborn: heart rate (HR), oxygen saturation (SPO2), color, screams, tonicity, reactivity.

The newborn behaviors have been modeled by means of six discrete states where State 0 is the "normal state" and State 5 is the death. The resulting newborn behaviors, for the ventilation gesture, are modeled by the state-chart diagram of the **Figure 11**.

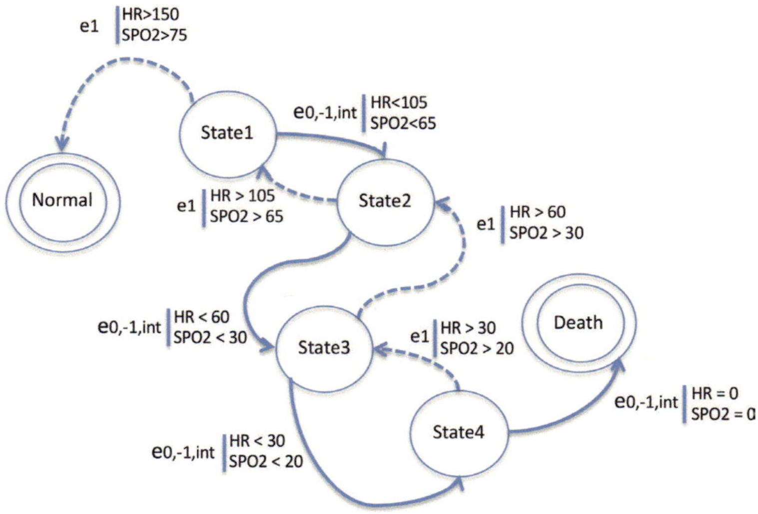

Figure 11.
State-chart diagram modeling the newborn's behavior according to the right or wrong execution of the ventilation gesture. $e_{0,-1,int}$ *is a shortened notation meaning that the degradation transition can be* e_0, e_{-1}, *or* e_{int}.

6. Conclusion

The chapter presents the methodology process implemented to develop a system of simulation to train medical practitioners to the resuscitation gestures. The process is based on building an application ontology used to elaborate conceptual models of the newborn behaviors and resuscitation gestures and to specify the system of simulation. The Manual Bag-Mask Ventilation gesture has been used to exemplify the implementation of the process. In the present state of realization, nasotracheal intubation and chest compression gestures have also been completely analyzed, modeled, and coded.

This work shows that the use of an application ontology is relevant to ensure the consistency of the modeling and specification processes since both use the same stabilized vocabulary. Furthermore, the ontology structures the domain (newborn resuscitation) according to the problem to solve (training medical staff) and to the problem solving method (simulation). The ontology was obtained through a cognitive approach, which consisted in applying the KOD method, which has proven to be adequate.

The simulation system including learners and professor management, simulation sessions, and debriefing sessions is performed. Three resuscitation gestures are currently available. Future works concern the development of the other resuscitation gestures as well as the final robot of the newborn.

Author details

Jean-Marc Mercantini
Data Processing and Systems Laboratory (Laboratoire d'Informatique et Systèmes - LIS UMR 7020), Domaine Universitaire de Saint Jérôme, CNRS, Aix-Marseille University, Toulon University, Marseille, France

*Address all correspondence to: jean-marc.mercantini@lis-lab.org

References

[1] Perlman JM, Willie J, Kattwinkel J, Wyckoff MH, Aziz K, Guinsburg R, et al. Part 7: Neonatal resuscitation: 2015 International Consensus on Cardiopulmonary Resuscitation and Emergency Cardiovascular Care Science With Treatment Recommendations. Pediatrics. 2015;**136**(Supplement 2): S120-S166

[2] Bétrémieux P. Prise en charge et réanimation du nouveau-né en salle de naissance: Synthèse, adaptation et commentaires pratiques des recommandations de l'International Liaison Committee on Resuscitation (ILCOR). Médecine et enfance. 2007;**27**:3-38. ISSN 0291-0233

[3] Silveira RC. Modélisation et conception d'un nouveau simulateur d'accouchement (BirthSim) pour l'entrainement et l'enseignement des jeunes obstétriciens et des sages femmes [thesis]. Institut National des Sciences Appliquées de Lyon (INSA); 2004

[4] Bimba AT, Idris N, Al-Hunaiyyan A, Mahmud RB, Abdelaziz A, Khan S, et al. Towards knowledge modelling and manipulation technologies: A survey. International Journal of Information Management. 2016;**36**:857-871

[5] Allert H, Markkanen H, Richter C. Rethinking the use of ontologies in learning. In: Tomadaki E, Scott P, editors. Proceedings of Innovative Approaches for Learning and Knowledge Sharing (EC-TEL). 2006. pp. 115-125. ISSN 1613-0073

[6] Wikipedia Dictionary [Internet]. 2018. Available from: http://en.wikipedia.org/wiki/Ontology

[7] ISCID. Encyclopedia of Science and Philosophy; International Society for Complexity, Information and Science [Internet]. 2008. Available from: http://www.iscid.org/encyclopedia/

[8] Gruber TR. Toward principles for the design of ontologies used for knowledge sharing. In: Technical Report KSL-93-04; Knowledge Systems Laboratory; Stanford University. 1993

[9] Gruber TR. Towards principles for the design of ontologies used for knowledge sharing. International Journal of Human-Computer Studies. 1995;**43**(5/6):907-928

[10] Uschold M, Grüninger M. Ontologies: Principles, methods and applications. Knowledge Engineering Review. 1996;**11**(2):93-136

[11] Guarino N. Semantic matching: Formal ontological distinctions for information organization, extraction, and integration. In: Pazienza MT, editor. Information Extraction: A Multidisciplinary Approach to an Emerging Information Technology. Springer Verlag; 1997. pp. 139-170

[12] Vandecasteele A. Modélisation Ontologique des Connaissances Expertes Pour L'analyse de Comportements à Risque : Application à la Surveillance Maritime. Économies et Finances. École Nationale Supérieure des Mines de Paris; 2012

[13] Vogel C. Génie Cognitif. Paris: Masson; 1988 (Sciences Cognitives)

[14] Mercantini JM, Tourigny N, Chouraqui E. Elaboration d'ontologies à partir de corpus en utilisant la méthode d'ingénierie des connaissances KOD. In: 1ère Édition des Journées Francophones sur les Ontologies (JFO); 18-20 Octobre 2007; Sousse, Tunisie. 2007. pp. 195-214. ISBN: 978-9973-37-414-1

[15] Dahlgren K. A linguistic ontology. International Journal of Human Computer Studies. 1995;**43**(5):809-818

[16] Fernández-López M. Overview of methodologies for building ontologies. In: Proceedings of the IJCAI-99 Workshop on Ontologies and Problem-Solving Methods (KRR5); 2 August, 1999; Stockhom;Sweden. pp. 4.1-4.13

[17] Aussenac-Gilles N, Biébow B, Szulman S. Revisiting ontology design: A method based on corpus analysis. In: Dieng R, Corby O, editors. Proceedings of the 12th International Conference on Knowledge Engineering and Knowledge Management (EKAW-2000); Springer-Verlag; LNAI. 1937. pp. 172-188

[18] Gandon F. Ontology engineering: A survey and a return on experience. In: Research Report No. 4396. INRIA; Sophia-Antipolis. 2002

[19] Sadok S, Chouraqui E, Mercantini JM. Modeling the deviation to improve safety aircraft piloting activities. In: Proceeding of the 1st IEE International Conference on System Safety; 6-8 June 2006; London. 2006

[20] Mercantini JM. Building a domain ontology to design a decision support software to plan fight actions against marine pollutions. In: Mercantini JM, Faucher C, editors. Risk and Cognition, Intelligent Systems Reference Library. Vol. 80. Springer-Verlag; 2015

[21] Sakli L, Mercantini JM, Hennet JC. Study of supply chain vulnerability based on cognitive engineering and ARIMA formal models. In: Proceeding of the 11th International Conference on Integrated Modelling and Analysis in Applied Control and Automation; 17-19 September 2018; Budapest. 2018

[22] Caroll JM. Chapter 17: Scenario-based design. In: Helander M, Landauer TK, Prabhu P, editors. Handbook of Human-Computer Interaction. 2nd ed. Amsterdam, North-Holland: Elsevier Science B.V; 1997

[23] Lavaud J, Ayachi A, editors. Réanimation et Transport Pédiatriques. 5th ed. Paris: Masson; 2004

Section 3

Treatment and Interventions

Chapter 6

The Importance of Lead Positioning to Improve Clinical Outcomes in Cardiac Resynchronization Therapy

Mirela-Anca Stoia, Sabina Istratoaie, Sorin Pop, Florin Anton, Sorin Crisan and Dan Blendea

Abstract

Left ventricular (LV) lead positioning is one of the main contributors to the cardiac resynchronization therapy (CRT) response. Conventional left ventricular (LV) lead implantation faces several difficulties, which may ultimately affect lead stability and performance. Several imaging techniques have been proposed to overcome all these obstacles including multimodality cardiac imaging to help in preprocedural or intraprocedural identification of the latest activated areas of the LV. Emerging pacing strategies like LV multisite and multipoint pacing may help deliver an enhanced response to CRT, but prospective trials are warranted to confirm the superiority of this approach.

Keywords: cardiac resynchronization therapy, left ventricular lead implant, coronary sinus, coronary venous tree, left bundle branch block

1. Introduction

Cardiac resynchronization therapy (CRT) exerts its physiological effect by restoring the atrioventricular, interventricular, and intraventricular synchronicity. This in turn results in an enhancement in pumping efficiency. In addition, CRT leads to an improved left ventricular (LV) filling and, in some cases, a reduction in the mitral regurgitation. The beneficial effects of CRT translate in a majority of patients in an improved quality of life, increased exercise capacity, reduction in hospitalization for heart failure, and reduction in overall mortality [1–3].

In spite of all these advantages, a substantial minority (approximately 30%) of patients treated with CRT do not show clinical improvement [3, 4]. The reasons for non-response to CRT include: lack of LV dyssynchrony, non-optimal position of the LV pacing lead, high-myocardial scar burden, and suboptimal device programming [5–10].

Given these considerations, the aim of this chapter was to review the different strategies of lead placement for CRT and their effect on clinical outcomes.

2. Coronary venous anatomy

2.1 The structure of the coronary venous tree

Lead positioning for CRT depends to a great extent on the coronary venous anatomy, which indirectly can impact outcomes of cardiac resynchronization.

The coronary sinus (CS) is a venous conduit situated in the vicinity of the left atrioventricular (AV) groove, which continues the great cardiac vein (GCV) and empties into the right atrium (**Figure 1**) [11]. Although the CS is a constant landmark vein, its length and diameter are highly variable. The diameter of the CS varies between 6 and 16 mm, while the diameter at its right atrial ostium can be from 5 to 20 mm. Its length can vary from 2 to 5 cm [11]. The major tributaries entering the CS-GCV are the anterior interventricular vein (AIV), the middle cardiac vein (MCV), the left marginal veins, and the posterolateral vein of the LV.

The AIV ascends in the anterior interventricular sulcus adjacent to the left anterior descending coronary artery from the apex toward the base of the heart. It then courses laterally at the base of the heart, along the left atrioventricular groove to form the GCV. This vein drains blood from the apical region of the heart, the anterior surfaces of both ventricles, and the anterior interventricular septum and parts of the left atrium [11]. The MCV travels along the inferior region of the heart, in the posterior interventricular groove, parallel to the posterior descending coronary artery [11]. The MCV drains the inferior walls of the ventricles, as well as the apical area and the posterior two-thirds of the septum. With an average diameter of 4 mm, the MCV empties into the CS near its right atrial ostium.

A more recent classification of the elements of the CS tree is the segmental approach, which, by establishing a correlation between venous tributaries and segments of the left ventricle, allows a more precise placement of the LV lead for enhancing cardiac synchrony [12]. The CS body is segmented along a horizontal axis, from the CS ostium to the anterior interventricular groove into three equal zones (**Figure 2**).

Branches originating in each segment are labeled posterior, lateral, or anterior segmental branches. The LV is divided along the longitudinal axis into three equal segments: basal, mid, and apical. The length of the first-degree tributaries and the position of the second-degree tributaries were defined according to these segments.

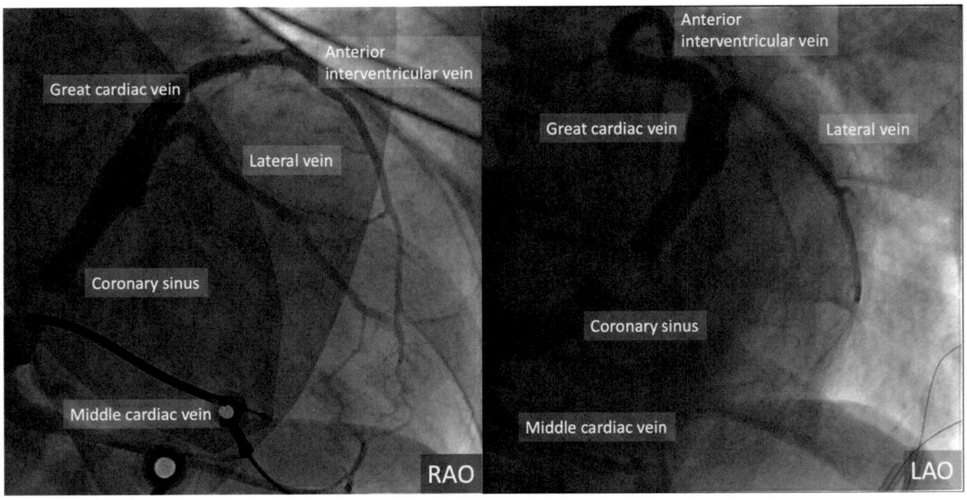

Figure 1.
The coronary venous tree as seen on a rotational angiogram.

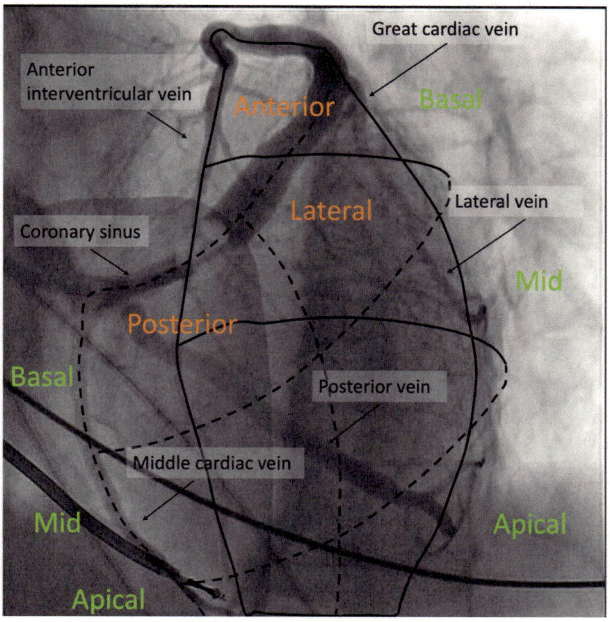

Figure 2.
Coronary venogram in the LAO view illustrating the segmental approach to venous anatomy. From the base to the apex, the heart is divided along the long axis into basal, mid, and apical segments. In this LAO projection, branches originating in each segment were labeled posterior, lateral, or anterior segmental branches. The length of the first-degree tributaries and the position of the second-degree tributaries were defined according to these segments.

This segmentation scheme also promotes potential optimization of the positioning of the LV lead along the lateral walls, framed by the network of second- and third-order branches—optimization that becomes necessary in the absence of a suitable first-order segmental branch.

In most patients undergoing CRT, the target veins used for LV lead placement include the posterior, posterolateral, and marginal veins of the left ventricle. The number of left posterior veins may be from one to three, but usually, it is a single vein (60%). It empties into the CS in 75% of cases, but it can also terminate in the GCV. There are a few cases with no left posterior vein (5%), giving the place to the left marginal vein to drain the left ventricular posterolateral wall [11]. Usually, the left marginal vein is a tributary of the GCV (81%), but in approximately 19% of cases, it can drain directly into the CS. It is also named the obtuse marginal vein and drains much of the left ventricular myocardium.

2.2 Coronary venous imaging

The electrophysiologist should be aware of both the usual geometry of the coronary venous tree and also of the common variants and the alterations in geometry induced by the underlying cardiac pathology. A clear appreciation of these variations by a careful pre-implantation planning may help position the LV lead in an optimal position and thus allow for successful CRT. Methods used for preprocedural evaluation of CV anatomy include multislice computed tomography (CT) [13], electron beam CT, and the levophase of coronary angiography.

A major disadvantage for CT in evaluation for CRT lies in the fact that it cannot be repeated during interventions, its role being limited to preprocedural evaluation. Another limit may be the difficulty in visualizing second- and third-order tributaries, details that are of paramount importance in optimal placing of the LV lead.

The most commonly used method of imaging to facilitate the LV lead placement is intraprocedural CV angiography [11]. This technique requires cannulation of the coronary sinus, and a balloon occlusion catheter is placed in the proximal CS to impede the flow of blood. The contrast material is then injected to opacify the CV tree by retrograde filling, thus enabling the delineation of the venous anatomy in real time.

Standard coronary venous angiography (SCVA) defines coronary venous anatomy in two orthogonal static views that may lead to suboptimal delineation of the origin, angulations, and course of the venous tributaries. When compared to standard venography, high-speed rotational coronary venous angiography (RCVA) offers a multi-angle dynamic view of the CV tree, providing a three-dimensional perspective [11]. As described previously, RCVA uses a rapid 4-second isocentric rotation of the imaging camera over a 110° arc from a right anterior oblique 55° to left anterior oblique 55° [11]. The rotational images can then be reviewed over a full range of angles, providing the operator with a superior assessment regarding the coronary venous tree and its branches than standard images. RCVA showed promising steps toward obtaining the desired imaging quality, providing multiple visualization angles, allowing for better identification, separation, and delimitation of the CS tree, all orders of segmental branches, as well as a more precise estimation of the take-off and angulation of its tributaries.

2.3 Variability of coronary venous anatomy in patients undergoing cardiac resynchronization therapy

During LV lead placement, knowledge of CS variations in morphology is of paramount importance as it may assist in the selection of the guiding catheter, leading to a successful CRT. The following anatomical features are important for CS cannulation: the CS ostial angle, the posterior displacement of the CS, the decrease in diameter at the junction between CS and great cardiac vein (GCV), the presence of stenoses and aneurysmal dilatations.

The CS ostial angle is acute in patients with severe tricuspid regurgitation and is more obtuse in patients with larger left atrial size [14].

While the CS is typically displaced from the left coronary sulcus toward the left atrium wall, the displacement is significantly more pronounced in patients post coronary artery bypass grafting (CABG) [15]. This, in turn, affects the shape of the GCV, accentuating its tortuosity, and thus, slowing or potentially stopping the advancement of the CS catheter during LV lead implant. Another potential obstruction of the CS cannulation may occur around the CS-GCV junction, in the form of a sudden diameter reduction in the area where the vein of Marshall takes off from the CS, as the latter continues as the GCV. The decrease in diameter of the vessel post junction appears to be greater in patients post CABG [15]. The intervention seems to also affect the probability of encountering stenoses and aneurysmal dilatations of the CS, which are encountered in 5–10% of cases, predominantly post CABG (**Figure 3**).

Current practice involves LV lead placement targeting mainly posterior or lateral veins. Indeed, a study that analyzed RVCA images of 51 patients undergoing CRT reported successful identification of lateral veins in 91% of the patients and posterior veins in 76% of cases [11]. However, in terms of suitability for LV lead placement, characteristics such as diameter and take-off angles render many of the identified branches suboptimal for implant. Both posterior and lateral veins were tortuous in 15–30% of the patients undergoing CRT implant [11].

Another factor affecting the placement of the LV lead is the presence of myocardial scar from prior myocardial infarctions (MIs). In a study by van de Veire et al., it

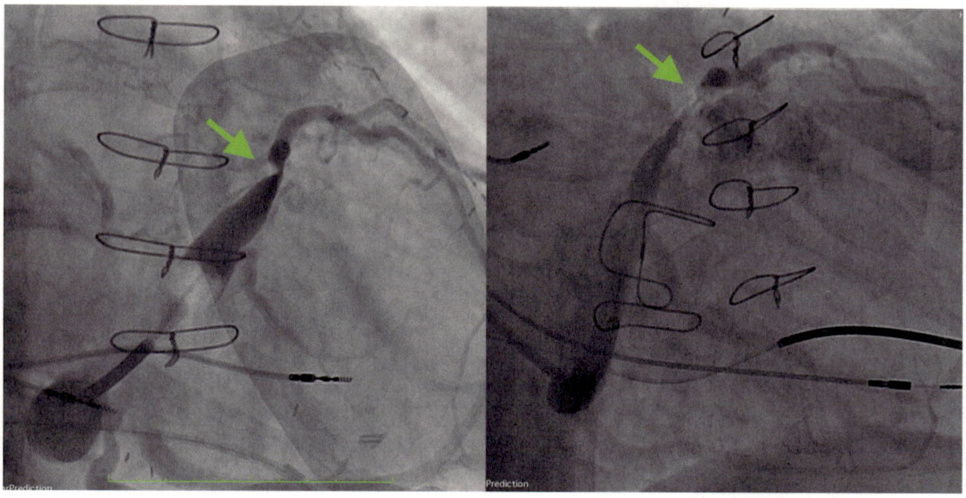

Figure 3.
Coronary sinus-great cardiac vein stenoses (green arrows) in patients with prior coronary artery bypass grafting.

was shown that patients with a history of myocardial infarction (MI) are less likely to CS tributaries in the segments with scar [13].

3. Electrical activation of the failing heart

3.1 Electrical activation in patients with left bundle branch block

Left bundle branch block (LBBB) can be associated with conduction delay located at several anatomic levels in the conduction system from the distal His bundle to the left bundle branch and further distally to the arborization of the left bundle branch system [3]. In patients with LBBB and heart failure, the first ventricular site to be activated is the right ventricular (RV) free wall. The activation then proceeds to the right septum, and the latest RV site to be activated is the posterobasal region [16]. The first sites of the LV to be activated vary, but, most often these are located in the apical septum, and more rarely in the septobasal or midseptal region or in the anterior wall [17, 18]. In most patients, the activation spreads around the apex and across the inferior wall, in a "U-shaped" pattern, and reaches the anterolateral wall of the LV and then progresses toward the basal posterior or posterolateral wall [3, 17, 18].

The endocardial activation encompasses about 75% of the duration of the QRS complex [16]. The rest of the QRS is represented by the activation of the mid-myocardium and epicardium [3, 18].

3.2 The electrical activation during CRT

During CRT, the RV and LV pacing leads generate two ventricular activation wavefronts, which move toward each other. If pacing is delivered with a sufficiently short AV delay, the left and right ventricular wavefronts merge before the intrinsic activation, conducted from the atria via the AV node, descends to the ventricles [3, 18–21]. The RV is depolarized entirely or almost entirely by the wavefront generated by the RV lead. The LV is activated from two sites: one situated in the interventricular septum initiated by the RV lead, and the other one situated onto the epicardial surface of the lateral LV initiated by the LV lead [17, 20, 22, 23].

4. Lead placement for cardiac resynchronization therapy

4.1 LV anatomical positioning: interlead distance

In order to implant an LV pacing lead via a transvenous approach, the CS is cannulated and the LV lead is advanced toward a second- or third-order branch of the CS situated preferably on the anterolateral, lateral, posterior, or posterolateral LV wall (**Figure 4**) [3, 10, 15, 18, 23].

Achieving maximal anatomical and electrical separation between the right and left ventricular leads [23] may have a beneficial impact on clinical outcomes [10, 18].

The significance of the anatomical interlead distance (**Figure 5**) was emphasized by Heist and colleagues [24] in a study on 51 consecutive patients referred for CRT. The Delta dp/dt value, measured by echo-Doppler, related to acute hemodynamic improvement was correlated with the corrected direct LV-RV horizontal interlead tips distance measured on postprocedural lateral radiographs. Acute hemodynamic responders to CRT (Delta dP/dt >25%) had higher corrected interlead distance on the lateral film in comparison with non-responders. The interlead distance was found to be a useful anatomic parameter to help in guiding the lead placement on LV and RV sites in order to optimize CRT outcomes [24].

4.2 Anatomical positioning: segmental pacing site

A commonly used CRT strategy involves the placement of the LV lead in an anatomically favorable position [25]. The usually targeted zones for LV lead implant are the basal to mid, lateral, or posterolateral LV areas, due to their most delayed onset of activation in patients with typical LBBB [25]. There is a general agreement that an apical lead position is less favorable [9, 26]. This was also shown in the Multicenter Automatic Defibrillator Implantation Trial-Cardiac Resynchronization Therapy (MADIT-CRT) [27].

Regarding the non-apical positions, the results in the literature are not always concordant. The REsynchronization reVErses Remodeling in Systolic Left vEntricular Dysfunction (REVERSE HF) trial revealed better outcomes with lateral lead placement [25, 28], while in the Comparison of Medical Therapy, Pacing, and

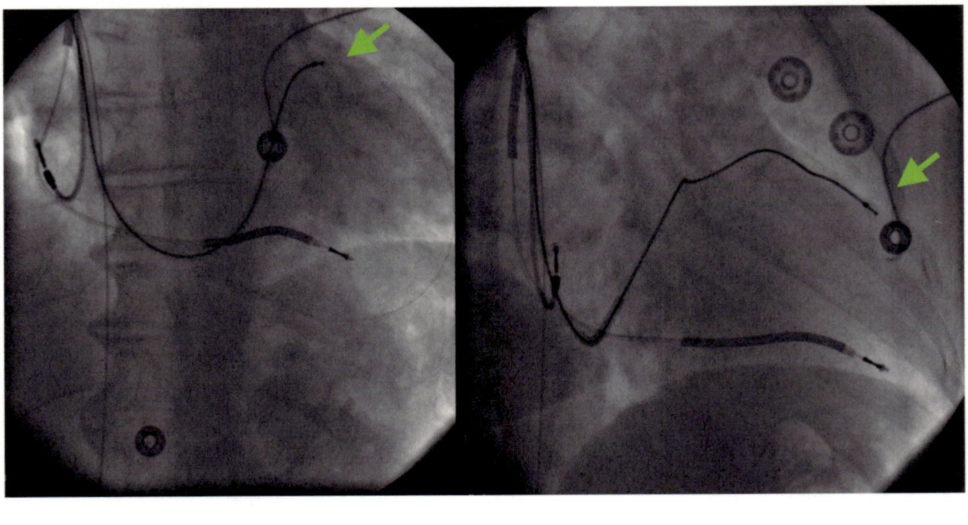

Figure 4.
Over-the-wire advancement of a left ventricular pacing lead into an anterolateral branch of the coronary sinus with final placement into a mid-ventricular segment.

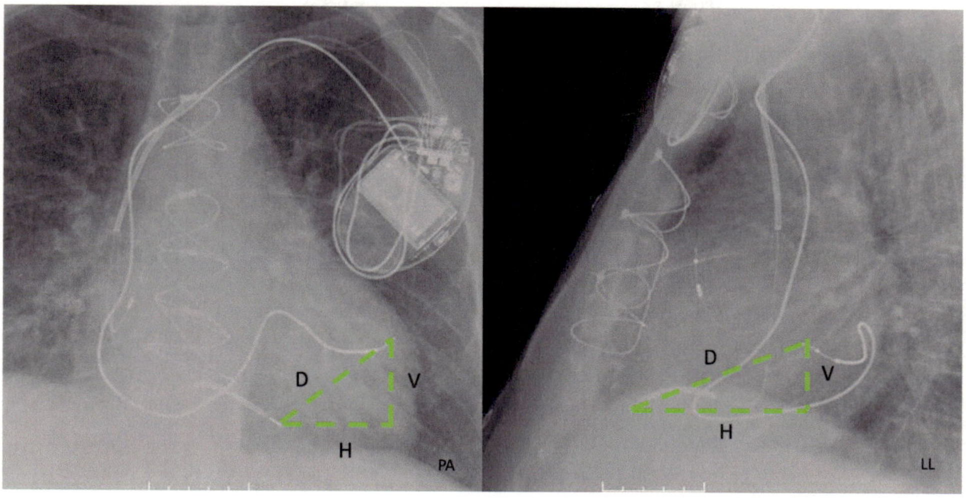

Figure 5.
Measurement of the interlead distance on the posteroanterior (PA) and lateral (LL) chest radiograph. D = interlead distance; H = horizontal dimension; V = vertical dimension.

Defibrillation in Heart Failure (COMPANION) trial and MADIT-CRT trial, the anterior, lateral, and posterior lead locations had comparable CRT outcomes [1].

Studies focused as well on a standardized anatomical positioning of LV lead implant according to its segmentation [12]. In the study by Merchant and colleagues [9], event-free survival was significantly lower in the patients with apical LV pacing, independent of clinical covariates. The apical group also demonstrated less improvement in NYHA functional class and less LV reverse remodeling. These data suggest that apical LV lead placement is associated with worse CRT outcomes and preferential positioning of LV leads in the basal/midventricle segments would be a choice in order to improve the outcomes. These results were also highlighted in a substudy analysis of the MADIT-CRT study [25, 29].

These observations have several potential explanations. Firstly, the LV depolarization wavefront in most conduction disturbances propagates from the apex to midventricle and last to the basal regions of the heart, which are the latest to be activated. Secondly, the main CRT objective is to synchronize the ventricles by electrical stimulation from RV and LV pacing sites, which ideally should be situated as far as possible from each other. An apically positioned LV lead is situated in the proximity of RV lead which results in reduced inter-electrode distance and inter-lead electrical separation, with unfavorable effects on heart failure evolution [18].

Besides anatomic segmental pacing position, shorter AV delays seem to increase the efficiency of LV apical pacing, as was shown in the article by Verbeek et al. [19]. Working on animal model, they demonstrated that LV function was optimized by using AV delays shorter than the baseline PQ time LV and BiV interconnected pacing, by excluding endogenous LV activation so far [18].

4.3 Maximum electrical delay

For an optimal result with cardiac resynchronization, it is necessary to detect the latest activated regions of LV, where the pacing lead should be preferably placed, resulting in LV hemodynamic improvements [18]. These LV areas of interest could be revealed by several invasive and non-invasive imaging techniques. One proposition was to use the intraprocedural measurement of the LV lead electrical delay

(LVLED), representing the calculated time between onset of the QRS on the surface ECG and the sensed signal on the LV lead (Q-LV) (**Figure 6**).

This delay is corrected for the baseline QRS (recorded simultaneously) by expressing it as a percentage of the baseline QRS duration (Q-LV/QRS duration ratio) [10].

Long LV lead electrical delays are linked with LV hemodynamic improvements, while shorter than 50% of LV lead electrical delays correlate with a worse clinical scenario [10, 18].

Both anatomic interlead separation and the LV electrical delay have been correlated with clinical outcomes following CRT in a study of Merchant and colleagues [9, 18]. They studied 61 consecutive patients undergoing CRT for standard clinical indications and found a positive correlation between corrected LVLED and horizontal interlead distance on lateral chest X-ray, and a negative correlation between LVLED and vertical interlead distance on posteroanterior chest X-ray [9, 18]. That inverse relationship has been transposed in a composite anatomic distance (defined as horizontal distance in lateral projection—vertical distance in PA projection), which correlated most closely with LVLED. These data suggest that LV-right ventricular interlead distance and LVED appear to synergistically combine anatomic and electrical parameters for predicting LV anatomic reverse remodeling and optimizing them means improving CRT outcomes [9, 18].

A retrospective study of Heist et al. that used a model that included anatomic, hemodynamic, and electrical data was able to accurately predict 12-month event-free survival [30].

Efforts are being made to further define the importance of the electrical delay strategy in implanting the LV lead. ENHANCE CRT is a trial that aims to compare

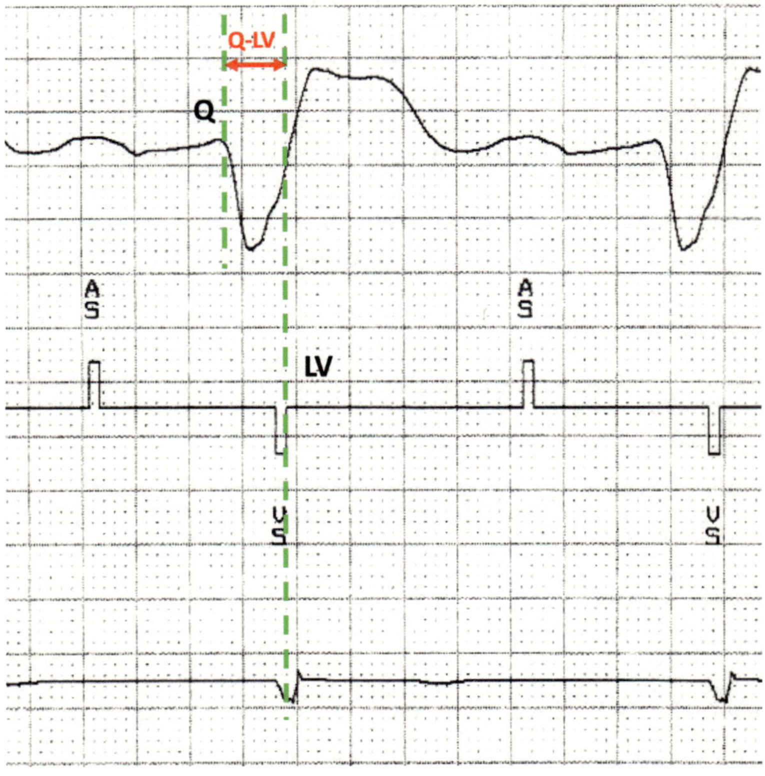

Figure 6.
Measurement of the Q-LV interval from the beginning of the QRS complex to the sensed electrogram on the left ventricular lead channel.

LV lead placement based on the electrical delay (Q-LV) with conventional implant in patients with non-LBBB [25, 31].

4.4 Maximum mechanical delay

Imaging techniques like tissue-Doppler, strain imaging, two-dimensional speckle-tracking imaging echocardiography, and tagged magnetic resonance imaging made possible identification of the latest activated segments of the LV [3, 6, 32, 33].

In a study on patients with heart failure undergoing CRT, that aimed to delineate the effects of CRT on LV performance, Ansalone et al. correlated the LV lead position with the site of the most mechanically delayed segment [6]. It was considered as concordance between LV pacing site and the most delayed area, when the LV lead was implanted in the region with the greatest regional mechanical delay as assessed by tissue Doppler. The results revealed that 42% of the patients were paced at a concordant site and showed the greatest improvements in clinical status and LV performance [3, 6].

A study evaluating the role of speckle-tracking echocardiography, an imaging modality that allows a more precise evaluation of the mechanical activation of different LV segments, revealed that LV lead implantation on the site of latest mechanical activation provided improvements in echocardiographic response after 6 months of CRT and better prognosis during long-term follow-up [33, 34].

Another study that assessed the impact of targeted LV lead placement using speckle-tracking echocardiography was the randomized targeted left ventricular lead placement to guide cardiac resynchronization therapy (TARGET) [35]. In the TARGET group of this study, the LV lead was positioned at the latest site of peak contraction with amplitude of 10% or greater to signify freedom from scar, while in the control group patients underwent standard CRT. When compared with controls, TARGET patients had a higher rate of lead concordance (lead placed at the most delayed LV segment) and higher rates of clinical response [35].

In the Speckle Tracking Assisted Resynchronization Therapy for Electrode Region (STARTER study), the concordance of LV lead with latest site was associated with an improvement in event-free survival [25, 36].

Summarizing the data available, there is no gold standard defined yet for selection of the optimal LV pacing segment and determination of the optimal pacing site could depend on input from several imaging modalities including image fusion strategies [25].

5. Emerging left ventricular pacing strategies

5.1 Endocardial pacing

During the electrical activation of epicardial pacing, the direction of pacing impulse is inverted, and that perturbation could become pro-arrhythmic. In this respect, endocardial biventricular pacing appears more physiological with the electrical impulse generated from endocardium and dissipated to epicardium [19]. The endocardial placement of LV lead is easier and without the restrictions of the coronary venous anatomy. Moreover, phrenic nerve stimulation could be often avoided, through the liberty to choose from multiple point LV lead positioning. The comparison with epicardial biventricular pacing seems to give encouraging results [19, 37–39].

Jais et al. [39] demonstrated that LV endocardial pacing is feasible. Other subsequent reports noticed improvement in clinical and of LV systolic function parameters [37, 40–43].

In an animal study on dogs with experimental LBBB, Van Deursen and colleagues [41] used pacing leads positioned in the right atrium, right ventricle, and at paired epicardial and endocardial LV sites. The endocardial biventricular pacing improved the electrical resynchronization and increased the benefit on LVdP/dt_{max} and stroke work by 90 and 50%, respectively, as compared with conventional epicardial approach [3]. Endocardial pacing seems not to be associated with the significant transmural dispersion of repolarization, often seen in epicardial procedures, and this in turn reduces the arrhythmogenic potential of CRT.

Another study that evaluated endocardial biventricular pacing [42] patients with ischemic cardiomyopathy revealed that endocardial biventricular pacing improved dP/dt(max) when compared with right ventricular apical pacing in all patients. In patients with pre-existing CS leads, LV endocardial pacing at the best endocardial site exceeded that achieved with the pre-implanted CRT device (using epicardial pacing via the existing CS lead). Optimal pacing sites were found to be located in LV segments outside from the postinfarct zone. The findings of this research suggest that CRT implanted at the best LV endocardial sites seems to be more effective than conventional CS lead epicardial pacing.

There are potential safety issues related to LV endocardial pacing such as thromboembolic complications or infection of the endocardial pacing lead [38]. Therefore, anticoagulation is required with a proposed international normalized ratio anticoagulation level around 3.5–4.5 (similar to mechanical valvular prostheses) [38].

5.2 Multisite and multipoint pacing

Another emerging LV pacing strategy is multisite pacing, which has been proposed as an alternative resynchronization strategy aimed at improving clinical and echocardiographic outcomes [44]. Triple-site pacing showed improved reverse remodeling and heart failure symptoms over a follow-up of 1 year, but implantation was shown to be difficult and the complication rate was higher than a standard approach [3, 45]. The Triple Resynchronization in Paced Heart Failure Patients (TRIP-HF) study of Leclercq et al. [44] compared the effects of triple-site versus dual-site biventricular pacing in 40 patients diagnosed with moderate-to-severe heart failure and permanent atrial fibrillation requiring cardiac pacing for slow ventricular rate. The results of this study showed that cardiac resynchronization therapy with one RV and two LV leads was associated with significantly more LV reverse remodeling than conventional biventricular stimulation.

Quadripolar leads renewed the interest in multipolar pacing. Pacing from the most proximal and distal individualized multipoint electrodes could lead to improved resynchronization [25, 46]. Multipoint pacing when compared with biventricular pacing was shown to be associated with improved ventricular systolic and diastolic parameters in an acute hemodynamic study [3, 47].

In a comparison between left ventricular endocardial, multisite, and multipolar epicardial pacing, the optimal pacing method was found to be individually specific, and on a group level, only endocardial pacing was superior to standard CRT from a hemodynamic standpoint [3, 48]. Within individuals, however, different methods of stimulation were found to be optimal, suggesting a need to tailor the pacing strategy to the underlying substrate [48].

Even though the results of multisite and multipoint pacing were not found to be consistently better than the conventional biventricular pacing modality, they remain an option for non-responders to conventional CRT, particularly for patients who have underlying myocardial scar and a more heterogeneous LV activation [49].

Further studies and prospective trials are warranted to help in identifying the subgroups of patients for whom the multisite pacing strategy provides clinical and hemodynamical results which are superior to standard CRT.

6. Conclusions

The last two decades have brought a multitude of technical developments in the field of CRT. However, the optimal strategy for left ventricular lead positioning, one of the most important factors that determine CRT outcomes, continues to remain poorly defined.

Anatomical positioning is currently the most frequently used LV lead implant strategy; however, several alternative approaches including targeting the most electrically or mechanically delayed region of the LV have been shown to be associated with superior CRT outcomes although the results have been variable. Further prospective studies are needed to better define a more reproducible and feasible technique for LV segment selection for CRT.

Conflict of interest

None.

Author details

Mirela-Anca Stoia[1], Sabina Istratoaie[1], Sorin Pop[1], Florin Anton[1], Sorin Crisan[2] and Dan Blendea[1,3]*

1 Emergency Clinical County Hospital, University of Medicine and Pharmacy "Iuliu Hatieganu", Cluj-Napoca, Romania

2 Municipal Clinical Hospital, University of Medicine and Pharmacy "Iuliu Hatieganu", Cluj-Napoca, Romania

3 Massachusetts General Hospital, Harvard Medical School, Boston, MA, USA

*Address all correspondence to: dblendea@me.com

References

[1] Bristow MR et al. Cardiac-resynchronization therapy with or without an implantable defibrillator in advanced chronic heart failure. The New England Journal of Medicine. 2004;**350**(21):2140-2150

[2] Cleland JG et al. The effect of cardiac resynchronization on morbidity and mortality in heart failure. The New England Journal of Medicine. 2005;**352**(15):1539-1549

[3] Blendea D, Singh JP. Lead positioning strategies to enhance response to cardiac resynchronization therapy. Heart Failure Reviews. 2011;**16**(3):291-303

[4] Abraham WT et al. Cardiac resynchronization in chronic heart failure. The New England Journal of Medicine. 2002;**346**(24):1845-1853

[5] Ypenburg C et al. Noninvasive imaging in cardiac resynchronization therapy—Part 2: Follow-up and optimization of settings. Pacing and Clinical Electrophysiology. 2008;**31**(12):1628-1639

[6] Ansalone G et al. Doppler myocardial imaging to evaluate the effectiveness of pacing sites in patients receiving biventricular pacing. Journal of the American College of Cardiology. 2002;**39**(3):489-499

[7] Bleeker GB et al. Postero-lateral scar tissue resulting in non-response to cardiac resynchronization therapy. Journal of Cardiovascular Electrophysiology. 2006;**17**(8):899-901

[8] Wilton SB et al. Relationship between left ventricular lead position using a simple radiographic classification scheme and long-term outcome with resynchronization therapy. Journal of Interventional Cardiac Electrophysiology. 2008;**23**(3):219-227

[9] Merchant FM et al. Impact of segmental left ventricle lead position on cardiac resynchronization therapy outcomes. Heart Rhythm. 2010;**7**(5):639-644

[10] Singh JP et al. Left ventricular lead electrical delay predicts response to cardiac resynchronization therapy. Heart Rhythm. 2006;**3**(11):1285-1292

[11] Blendea D et al. Variability of coronary venous anatomy in patients undergoing cardiac resynchronization therapy: A high-speed rotational venography study. Heart Rhythm. 2007;**4**(9):1155-1162

[12] Singh JP et al. The coronary venous anatomy: A segmental approach to aid cardiac resynchronization therapy. Journal of the American College of Cardiology. 2005;**46**(1):68-74

[13] Van de Veire NR et al. Non-invasive visualization of the cardiac venous system in coronary artery disease patients using 64-slice computed tomography. Journal of the American College of Cardiology. 2006;**48**(9):1832-1838

[14] Blendea D et al. Impact of tricuspid regurgitation and prior coronary bypass surgery on the geometry of the coronary sinus: A rotational coronary angiography study. Journal of Cardiovascular Electrophysiology. 2010;**21**(4):436-440

[15] Blendea D, Altman RK, Singh JP. Procedural aspects of lead positioning for cardiac resynchronization therapy. The Journal of Innovations in Cardiac Rhythm Management. 2011;**2**:165-171

[16] Rodriguez LM et al. Variable patterns of septal activation in patients with left bundle branch block and

heart failure. Journal of Cardiovascular Electrophysiology. 2003;**14**(2):135-141

[17] Auricchio A et al. Characterization of left ventricular activation in patients with heart failure and left bundle-branch block. Circulation. 2004;**109**(9):1133-1139

[18] Ellenbogen KA, Auricchio A. American Heart Association. Pacing to Support the Failing Heart. AHA Clinical Series. Chichester, UK; Hoboken, NJ: Wiley-Blackwell; 2008. xiii. 347 p

[19] Verbeek XA et al. Intra-ventricular resynchronization for optimal left ventricular function during pacing in experimental left bundle branch block. Journal of the American College of Cardiology. 2003;**42**(3):558-567

[20] Jia P et al. Electrocardiographic imaging of cardiac resynchronization therapy in heart failure: Observation of variable electrophysiologic responses. Heart Rhythm. 2006;**3**(3):296-310

[21] Lambiase PD et al. Non-contact left ventricular endocardial mapping in cardiac resynchronisation therapy. Heart. 2004;**90**(1):44-51

[22] Prinzen FW, Spinelli JC, Auricchio A. Basic physiology and hemodynamics of cardiac pacing. In: Ellenbogen KA et al., editors. Clinical Cardiac Pacing, Defibrillation, and Resynchronization Therapy. Philadelphia PA, USA: Saunders; 2007. pp. 291-335

[23] Singh JP et al. Dialing-in cardiac resynchronization therapy: Overcoming constraints of the coronary venous anatomy. Journal of Interventional Cardiac Electrophysiology. 2006;**17**(1):51-58

[24] Heist EK et al. Radiographic left ventricular-right ventricular interlead distance predicts the acute hemodynamic response to cardiac resynchronization therapy. The American Journal of Cardiology. 2005;**96**(5):685-690

[25] Roka A, Borgquist R, Singh J. Coronary sinus lead positioning. Heart Failure Clinics. 2017;**13**(1):79-91

[26] Brignole M et al. ESC guidelines on cardiac pacing and cardiac resynchronization therapy: The task force on cardiac pacing and resynchronization therapy of the European Society of Cardiology (ESC). Developed in collaboration with the European Heart Rhythm Association (EHRA). The European Heart Journal. 2013;**34**(29):2281-2329

[27] Singh JP et al. Left ventricular lead position and clinical outcome in the multicenter automatic defibrillator implantation trial-cardiac resynchronization therapy (MADIT-CRT) trial. Circulation. 2011;**123**(11):1159-1166

[28] Linde C et al. Randomized trial of cardiac resynchronization in mildly symptomatic heart failure patients and in asymptomatic patients with left ventricular dysfunction and previous heart failure symptoms. Journal of the American College of Cardiology. 2008;**52**(23):1834-1843

[29] Kutyifa V et al. Left ventricular vead location and long-term outcomes in cardiac resynchronization therapy patients. JACC: Clinical Electrophysiology. Nov 2018;**4**(11):1410-1420

[30] Heist EK et al. Usefulness of a novel "response score" to predict hemodynamic and clinical outcome from cardiac resynchronization therapy. The American Journal of Cardiology. 2006;**97**(12):1732-1736

[31] Singh JP et al. Rationale and design for enhance CRT: QLV implant strategy for non-left bundle branch

block patients. ESC Heart Fail. 2018;**5**(6):1184-1190

[32] Lardo AC, Abraham TP, Kass DA. Magnetic resonance imaging assessment of ventricular dyssynchrony: Current and emerging concepts. Journal of the American College of Cardiology. 2005;**46**(12):2223-2228

[33] Ypenburg C et al. Optimal left ventricular lead position predicts reverse remodeling and survival after cardiac resynchronization therapy. Journal of the American College of Cardiology. 2008;**52**(17):1402-1409

[34] Becker M et al. Impact of left ventricular lead position on the efficacy of cardiac resynchronisation therapy: A two-dimensional strain echocardiography study. Heart. 2007;**93**(10):1197-1203

[35] Khan FZ et al. Targeted left ventricular lead placement to guide cardiac resynchronization therapy: The TARGET study: A randomized, controlled trial. Journal of the American College of Cardiology. 2012;**59**(17):1509-1518

[36] Saba S et al. Echocardiography-guided left ventricular lead placement for cardiac resynchronization therapy: Results of the speckle tracking assisted resynchronization therapy for electrode region trial. Circulation. Heart Failure. 2013;**6**(3):427-434

[37] Garrigue S et al. Comparison of chronic biventricular pacing between epicardial and endocardial left ventricular stimulation using Doppler tissue imaging in patients with heart failure. The American Journal of Cardiology. 2001;**88**(8):858-862

[38] van Gelder BM et al. Transseptal endocardial left ventricular pacing: An alternative technique for coronary sinus lead placement in cardiac resynchronization therapy. Heart Rhythm. 2007;**4**(4):454-460

[39] Jais P et al. Mid-term follow-up of endocardial biventricular pacing. Pacing and Clinical Electrophysiology. 2000;**23**(11 Pt 2):1744-1747

[40] Garrigue S et al. Usefulness of biventricular pacing in patients with congestive heart failure and right bundle branch block. The American Journal of Cardiology. 2001;**88**(12):1436-1441, A8

[41] van Deursen C et al. Left ventricular endocardial pacing improves resynchronization therapy in canine left bundle-branch hearts. Circulation. Arrhythmia and Electrophysiology. 2009;**2**(5):580-587

[42] Spragg DD et al. Optimal left ventricular endocardial pacing sites for cardiac resynchronization therapy in patients with ischemic cardiomyopathy. Journal of the American College of Cardiology. 2010;**56**(10):774-781

[43] Bordachar P et al. Left ventricular endocardial stimulation for severe heart failure. Journal of the American College of Cardiology. 2010;**56**(10):747-753

[44] Leclercq C et al. A randomized comparison of triple-site versus dual-site ventricular stimulation in patients with congestive heart failure. Journal of the American College of Cardiology. 2008;**51**(15):1455-1462

[45] Rogers DP et al. A randomized double-blind crossover trial of triventricular versus biventricular pacing in heart failure. European Journal of Heart Failure. 2012;**14**(5): 495-505

[46] Thibault B et al. Acute haemodynamic comparison of multisite and biventricular pacing with a quadripolar left ventricular lead. Europace. 2013;**15**(7):984-991

[47] Pappone C et al. Multipoint left ventricular pacing improves acute hemodynamic response assessed with pressure-volume loops in cardiac resynchronization therapy patients. Heart Rhythm. 2014;**11**(3):394-401

[48] Shetty AK et al. A comparison of left ventricular endocardial, multisite, and multipolar epicardial cardiac resynchronization: An acute haemodynamic and electroanatomical study. Europace. 2014;**16**(6):873-879

[49] Niederer SA et al. Biophysical modeling to simulate the response to multisite left ventricular stimulation using a quadripolar pacing lead. Pacing and Clinical Electrophysiology. 2012;**35**(2):204-214

Chapter 7

Public-Access Defibrillation in Sudden Cardiac Arrest

Ruslan Linchak, Sergey Boytsov, Andrey Ardashev and Artem Kuzovlev

Abstract

Sudden cardiac arrest caused by cardiac and extracardiac pathology is one of the leading causes of death in developed countries. Public-access defibrillation is one of the key techniques for improvement of the pre-hospital and in-hospital resuscitation success and survival rates of resuscitated patients in the case of a sudden cardiac arrest caused by ventricular fibrillation and pulseless ventricular tachycardia. This book chapter will discuss the relation between the type of a sudden cardiac arrest and the survival rate and the "chain of survival" concept and the role of early public-access defibrillation, as well as the function of public-access defibrillation programs and the contribution of automated external defibrillators in pre-hospital and in-hospital resuscitation.

Keywords: cardiac arrest, cardiopulmonary resuscitation, chain of survival, public-access defibrillation

1. Introduction

Sudden cardiac arrest (SCA) caused by cardiac and extracardiac pathologies is one of the leading causes of death in the developed countries [1]. Mechanisms of SCA development are as follows: (a) ventricular fibrillation (VF) and pulseless ventricular tachycardia (PVT), shockable rhythms, and (b) asystole (As) and pulseless electrical activity (PEA), non-shockable rhythms.

2. Pre-hospital sudden cardiac arrest

In the United States, pre-hospital SCA develops approximately in 350,000 people per year. In Russia, 200,000–250,000 patients suddenly die from heart diseases every year. In most European countries, an average of approximately 87 cases of SCA per 100,000 people was registered every year before 2010; 84 cases were registered from 2011 to 2015 [2, 3]. Over the past 25 years, a progressive decrease in the incidence of VF was observed, which to a certain extent is related to the primary and secondary prevention of heart diseases and SCA.

The time of registration (diagnosis) of SCA is crucial. For example, in the case of a prolonged (>5–8 min) pre-hospital cardiac arrest, VF before the start of cardiopulmonary resuscitation (CPR) was registered only in 25% (20–40%) of patients. However, if ECG was registered within the first minutes of the SCA at public places equipped with an automated external defibrillators (AED), VF was registered in 49–76% [4, 5]. Data of the analysis of the cardiac rhythm carried out from 2006 to 2012 demonstrated that 25–50% of SCA resulted from VF and PVT [1, 6, 7]. According to two multicenter studies carried out in the United States and Europe from 2011 to 2015, VF and PVT were registered in 15.5 and 12.5–22%, respectively [3, 8]. The survival rate of resuscitated patients with pre-hospital VF/PVT in various regions of Canada and the United States before 2010 ranged from 7.7 to 40% (median 22%), while the overall survival after all kinds of pre-hospital SCA (As, PEA, VF/PVT) ranged only from 3 to 12.6% (median 8.4%) [9]. In the European studies, the survival rate in VF/PVT in Denmark increased from 16.3 to 35.7% and in As/PEA from 0.6 to 1.8% over the period from 2005 to 2012 [10]. In the Netherlands over the specified time period, the survival rate increased only in the case of VF/PVT (from 29 to 41.4%); in the case of the development of As/PEA, it remained nearly unchanged (3.1–2.7%) [6].

According to the recent studies (2011–2015) in five US states, the survival rate in all kinds of SCA (n = 65,000) averaged 11.4% (the range by states varied from 8.0 to 16.1%); in VF/PVT it was 34% (varied depending on the state from 26.4 to 44.7%). In 27 European countries (2014), the survival rate in all kinds of SCA (n = 10,600) amounted to 10.7% (by countries: from <5 to 31%), after the primary VF, it was 29.7% (by countries: from 5.3 to 58%), and after all the cases of primary and secondary, it was on average 21% [3, 8].

2.1 Sudden cardiac arrest at home

According to Weisfeldt et al. [5], if the AED was available to the first witness of a home cardiac arrest, VF/PVT was registered in 36% of cases and in 25% of cases if CPR was started by the staff of the emergency medical service (EMS). In that case the survival rate was on average 12% (2.8 times less than the number of resuscitated patients at public places equipped with the AEDs). The causes of such a low survival rate after CPR at home were apparently as follows: (a) frequent unwitnessed SCA, (b) frequent lack of the AED for the first witness of the SCA, and (c) small incidence of SCA caused by a cardiac pathology (primary SCA) [1, 11].

3. In-hospital cardiac arrest

According to two studies (1999–2005) in hospitals in the United States and several European countries, the primary VF/PVT was registered in 24–35% of patients; the survival rate in this study [12] was an average of 37%, and in the study [13] it ranged from 18 to 67%. In the study [14] it was found that in the United States, the incidence of the in-hospital VF/PVT decreased from 23.5 to 18.5% over the period from 2000 to 2009; while the survival rate increased from 28 to 39%. When the primary As and PEA developed (about 70% of all SCA cases), the survival rate was on average 11 and 12%, respectively (ranged from 1.2 to 14%) [12, 13]. It was also noticed that during CPR in approximately 20% of patients with the primary As or secondary PEA (i.e., terminal), VF/PVT develops; this combination was associated with a reduced survival rate. For instance, in the case of the primary As with the development of the secondary VF/PVT during the CPR, the survival rate was 8% (without secondary VF/PVT it was 12%), and with the primary PEA, it was 7% (without secondary VF/PVT it was 14%) [12].

In the studies conducted in Norway from 2009 to 2013, the in-hospital primary VF/PVT was registered in 27–32% of patients; As was found in 19–23% and PEA in 48% of patients. The survival rate of patients with VF/PVT amounted to 53% and in patients with cardiac pathology it was 61%; the survival rate in the case of As was 17%, in the case of PEA it was 13%, and the overall survival was 25% [15, 16]. In the UK (data analyzed from 2011 to 2013 in 144 hospitals) the VF/PVT caused SCA in 17% of patients, As in 23.6% of patients, and PEA in 49% of patients; the survival rate was 49% for VF/PVT, 8.7% for As, and 11.4% for PEA, and the overall survival was 18.4% [17]. In Italy (data analyzed from 2012 to 2014 in 36 hospitals) VF/PVT was registered in 19% of patients; the overall survival rate was 14.8% [18].

Therefore, both pre-hospital and in-hospital SCA caused by the primary VF/PVT, unlike the SCA caused by the primary As and PEA, are characterized by significantly higher survival rates of resuscitated patients. Analysis of the data from international studies published from 1990 to 2005 showed that if CPR during a prolonged SCA was initiated 5–8 min after the onset of SCA, the overall survival rate was on average 6.4%. However, if the pre-hospital CPR and AED are conducted within the first 3–5 min after the onset of SCA by trained personnel (non-health-care workers), the survival rate can reach up to 74–49%. These data were obtained when AEDs were placed in airports, airplanes, and casinos. This high survival rate was provided by the introduction of the "chain of survival" concept and the program of immediate start of basic CPR and rapid application of the AED. It should be noted that in cases of development of VF or PVT, each minute of delay of the CPR start reduces the probability of the survival by 7–10% and delay of the defibrillation by 10–15%. Unfortunately, even in the leading European countries, rapid start of CPR by an accidental witness of the SCA was undertaken only in one third of cases, and basic CPR with AED was carried out even more rarely. In this regard the main objective of the 2005–2010 international CPR guidelines as well as changes in educational materials was to increase the survival rate due to earlier and high-quality basic CPR with an extensive use of the AEDs [4, 19–21].

It should be noted that the causes of low survival rates after pre-hospital SCA are more difficult to study with evidence-based medicine methods. Many studies have focused on short-term outcomes of CPR: return of spontaneous circulation and short-term survival. However, the main criteria of successful pre-hospital resuscitation are long-term results, i.e., survival to discharge and survival and quality of life within 1–5 years after SCA (long-term survival).

4. The chain of survival concept

4.1 The "chain of survival"

The "chain of survival" concept was formulated by the experts of the American Heart Association in the early 1990s. According to this concept, the success of CPR and the survival rate of patients with pre-hospital SCA may be increased if the following criteria are met: early recognition and call for help, early bystander CPR, early defibrillation, early advanced life support, and standardized post-resuscitation care. In this case, the survival rate can be increased by more than twofold [22, 23]. Delay in any step of the chain of survival leads to a deterioration of the CPR results and reduction of the survival rates [5–7].

When heart rate monitoring is not available, SCA is diagnosed within no more than 10 s by means of the following clinical signs: unconsciousness, no normal breathing or agonal breathing, and no pulse on the carotid artery. Within the first minutes after SCA, the agonal respiration develops in 40% of the victims. Sudden cardiac arrest can in the beginning cause a short convulsive episode (seizures) which can be mistaken for epilepsy. The final changes in skin color, most often pallor or cyanosis, are not diagnostic for SCA [1].

After the diagnosis of SCA, the local EMS should be notified immediately (at the pre-hospital stage, ambulance service, and in-hospital, anaesthesiologists and intensivists), and CPR should be started with chest compressions of appropriate quality. In most countries of the world, the average time from a call to the EMS service before it arrives in place is 5–8 min. During this time the patient's survival depends on the CPR and AED providers [1, 5–11].

Immediate start of chest compressions increases survival in SCA by 2–3 times. Chest compressions and defibrillation performed within 3–5 min from the development of SCA provide survival rate of 49–75%. Every minute of delay with defibrillation reduces the likelihood of survival by 10–15%. Early defibrillation is possible if an AED located in a public place is available [1, 5–11].

4.2 Quality of cardiopulmonary resuscitation

In the European Resuscitation Council Guidelines for Resuscitation 2015 [1, 4], the reference criteria for the quality of chest compressions are the following: hand position on the center of the chest; rate 100–120 per minute with as few interruptions as possible; depth at least 5 cm, but not more than 6 cm; allow the chest to recoil completely after each compression; and do not lean on the chest. Chest compression fraction (the percentage of time from the total time of CPR spent only for chest compression) should be at least 60% of the total time of CPR. Pauses in chest compressions should be no more than 10 s for mouth-to-mouth ventilations and no more than 5 s for defibrillation. Hyperventilation should be avoided during CPR (recommended ventilation rate—10–12 breaths/min) since it leads to an increase in intrathoracic pressure, a decrease in coronary perfusion pressure, and an increase in mortality rate.

There is evidence that chest compression depth range of 4.5–5.5 cm in adults leads to better outcomes (survival-to-discharge) than all other compression depths during manual CPR [24–26]. Compression depth of more than 6 cm is associated with an increased rate of injury in adults when compared with compression depths of 5–6 cm during manual CPR [27]. A higher survival rate (survival-to-discharge) was found among patients who received chest compressions at a rate of 100–120/min, compared to >140/min and 120–139/min [28, 29]. The low chest compression release velocity (CCRV) worsens the outcome of CPR: the odds ratios for survival for CCRV ≥400 mm/s and 300–399.9 mm/s was 4.17 and 3.08, respectively; CCRV ≥400 mm/s was associated with a higher rate of favorable neurological outcomes; an increase in the CCRV for every 10 mm/s was associated with an increase in the survival rate [30, 31]. Our data [Kuzovlev et al., 2018; unpublished] show that during the in-hospital CPR, the quality of chest compressions was extremely low (rate 124.9 ± 22.3/min; depth 4.6 ± 1.1 cm; chest compressions in target 5.4 ± 18.3%; CCRV 324.5 ± 93.5 mm/s), but it significantly improved with feedback devices (rate 111.9 ± 7.3/min; depth 5.2 ± 0.4 cm; chest compressions in target 68.3 ± 26.4%; CCRV 352.1 ± 40.2 mm/s). CCRV was moderate and did not improve with feedback devices.

5. Early defibrillation concept

In 1991 the American Heart Association experts formulated the concept of early defibrillation. According to this concept, early defibrillation is the most important link in the chain of survival: in the hospital, it must be performed within the first 2–3 min of SCA and within 3–5 min during the pre-hospital stage. The main principle of early defibrillation is that the first rescuers arriving to the patient should have the AED; if it is not available, manual defibrillator should be available [1, 4].

6. Public-access defibrillation concept

A wide use of the AED outside the hospital by minimally trained personnel without medical education formed the basis of the concept of public-access defibrillation, which was formulated by the American Heart Association experts in 1994. Based on this concept, programs of the pre-hospital use of the AED by the first SCA witnesses were developed in the United States and Europe. According to studies published in 2010–2016, use of the AED by the first responders caused by the primary VF/PVT significantly increases the number of survivors to discharge [6, 32–35]. Therefore, a wide use of AEDs can improve outcomes in the pre-hospital SCA. However, AEDs are not frequently used in a number of European countries. For example, according to Agerskov et al. [33], in Denmark, the first responders of SCA applied the AED before the EMS arrival only in 3.8% of patients.

7. Public-access defibrillation (PAD) programs

Public-access defibrillation programs include a number of elements: contact with a local EMS, location of the AED and criteria for its selection, and principles and quality of training in basic CPR/AED.

7.1 Contact with a local emergency medicine service and its dispatcher

The European Resuscitation Council Guidelines for Resuscitation 2015 [1, 4] emphasize the essential role of interactions between an EMS dispatcher and basic CPR and AED providers. The dispatcher plays an important role in the early diagnosis of SCA and starting of high-quality CPR (the so-called telephone-assisted CPR), as well as in searching for the AED and ensuring its delivery to the scene [1, 36]. Organization of cardiac arrest centers and their contacts with regional and local EMS should be encouraged because it is associated with an increase in the survival rates and improvement of neurological outcomes in patients with pre-hospital cardiac arrest [1].

7.2 Location of the AED and criteria for its selection

There are several criteria for selection of the AED location. Time factor is one of the most significant criteria. It is economically feasible to place the AEDs in those public places where one SCA may be expected once per 5 years [1, 3]. According to the European Resuscitation Council experts, the ideal location for the AED must be at such a distance that a first responder could spend no more than 1.5 min to take it and return back to the patient. In this case an EMS dispatcher can help the provider to locate the AED. For this purpose it is necessary to register AEDs located in public areas. According to M. Agerskov et al. [33], in Denmark, only 15% of all SCA cases were registered within 100 meters from the location of the AED.

7.3 Training in basic CPR/AED

It is noteworthy that in the case of the pre-hospital cardiac arrest caused by VF, early high-quality chest compressions and defibrillation are key factors to the success of the resuscitation and survival [1, 4]. According to [37, 38] effective training of nonprofessionals in the basic CPR/AED increases the long-term survival (by the 30th day and 1 year of observation). It was also shown that well-trained EMS managers were able to improve CPR carried out by first responders [1, 39, 50].

8. In-hospital public-access defibrillation

Worldwide, depending on the model of the device, in-hospital AEDs are used in three modes: semiautomatic, fully automatic, and manual. Semiautomatic and, less frequently, manual modes are used in PAD. It should be noted that there are still no results from randomized clinical trials comparing the use of the hospital manual defibrillators and the AED in semiautomatic mode. At the same time, three observational studies were conducted which detected no increase in survival rates using the AED [40–42], and one study even demonstrated its decrease as compared with the use of manual defibrillators [43]. The results of study [44] suggest that the AED use may delay the start of the basic CPR and increase the duration of pauses in chest compressions which can be deleterious in SCA related to non-shockable rhythms (primary asystole and PEA, when defibrillation is contraindicated).

Based on the results, the European Resuscitation Council experts (2015) recommend to use the AED in the semiautomatic mode in those hospitals units where there is a risk of delay in defibrillation for a few minutes (more than 2–3 min) and the first responders have no experience in manual defibrillation. In those hospital units where quick access to manual defibrillators can be provided, manual defibrillation should be conducted either by trained medical personnel or the resuscitation team—this is preferred to the use of the AED because it reduces the time from the onset of the SCA to the first shock. However, in such cases, experience in the visual analysis of the electrocardiogram (ECG) is required [1, 50]. The European Resuscitation Council Guidelines for Resuscitation 2015 for the use of automatic and manual defibrillators for the PAD are based on the studies conducted in the United States and Australia [40–50]. It should be however noted that no similar studies were conducted in Russia; therefore, at present time, this recommendation can be introduced in the practice of those Russian hospitals which have special resuscitation teams and/or trained staff experienced in a fast analysis of ECG and work with manual defibrillators.

9. Conclusion

Sudden cardiac arrest caused by cardiac and extracardiac pathology is one of the leading causes of death in developed countries. The success of CPR and the survival rate of patients with pre-hospital SCA may be increased if the following criteria are met: early recognition and call for help, early bystander CPR, early defibrillation, early advanced life support, and standardized post-resuscitation care. In this case, the survival rate can be increased by more than two-fold. Public-access defibrillation is one of key techniques for improvement of the pre-hospital and in-hospital resuscitation success and survival rates of resuscitated patients in the case of a SCA caused by ventricular fibrillation and pulseless ventricular tachycardia.

Conflict of interest

None.

Notes/thanks/other declarations

None.

DOI: http://dx.doi.org/10.5772/intechopen.80607

Author details

Ruslan Linchak[1], Sergey Boytsov[2], Andrey Ardashev[3] and Artem Kuzovlev[4]*

1 National Medical Research Center for Preventive Medicine, Moscow, Russia

2 National Medical Research Center for Cardiology, Moscow, Russia

3 Department of Arrhythmias, Medical Research and Education Center, M.V. Lomonosov Moscow State University, Moscow, Russia

4 Federal Research and Clinical Center of Intensive Care Medicine and Rehabilitology, V.A. Negovsky Research Institute of General Reanimatology, Moscow, Russia

*Address all correspondence to: artem_kuzovlev@mail.ru

References

[1] Moroz VV, editor. The 2015 European Resuscitation Council Guidelines for Resuscitation. 3rd ed. Moscow: NIIOR, RusNRC; 2016. p. 192

[2] Benjamin EJ, Blaha MJ, Chiuve SE, Cushman M, Das SR, Deo R, et al. Heart disease and stroke statistics—2017 update: A report from the American Heart Association. Circulation. 2017;**135**(10):e146-e603. DOI: 10.1161/CIR.0000000000000485

[3] Gräsner JT, Lefering R, Koster RW, Masterson S, Böttiger BW, Herlitz J, et al. EuReCa ONE-27 Nations, ONE Europe, ONE Registry: A prospective one month analysis of out-of-hospital cardiac arrest outcomes in 27 countries in Europe. Resuscitation. 2016;**105**:188-195. DOI: 10.1016/j.resuscitation.2016.06.004

[4] Handley AJ, Koster R, Monsieurs K, Perkins GD, Davies S, Bossaert L, et al. European Resuscitation Council guidelines for resuscitation 2005. Section 2. Adult basic life support and use of automated external defibrillators. Resuscitation. 2005;**67**(Suppl 1):S7-S23. DOI: 10.1016/j.resuscitation.2005.10.007

[5] Weisfeldt ML, Everson-Stewart S, Sitlani C, Rea T, Aufderheide TP, Atkins DL, et al. Ventricular tachyarrhythmias after cardiac arrest in public versus at home. The New England Journal of Medicine. 2011;**364**(4):313-321. DOI: 10.1056/NEJMoa1010663

[6] Blom MT, Beesems SG, Homma PC, Zijlstra JA, Hulleman M, van, Hoeijen DA, et al. Improved survival after out-of-hospital cardiac arrest and use of automated external defibrillators. Circulation. 2014;**130**:1868-1875. DOI: 10.1161/CIRCULATIONAHA.114.010905

[7] Hulleman M, Berdowski J, de Groot JR, van, Dessel PF, Borleffs CJ, Blom MT, et al. Implantable cardioverter-defibrillators have reduced the incidence of resuscitation for out-of-hospital cardiac arrest caused by lethal arrhythmias. Circulation. 2012;**126**:815-821. DOI: 10.1161/CIRCULATIONAHA.111.089425

[8] van, Diepen S, Girotra S, Abella BS, Becker LB, Bobrow BJ, Chan PS, et al. Multistate 5-year initiative to improve care for out-of-hospital cardiac arrest: Primary results from the Heart Rescue Project. Journal of the American Heart Association. 2017;**6**(9):e005716. DOI: 10.1161/JAHA.117.005716

[9] Nichol G, Thomas E, Callaway CW, Hedges J, Powell JL, Aufderheide TP, et al. Regional variation in out-of-hospital cardiac arrest incidence and outcome. JAMA. 2008;**300**(12):1423-1431. DOI: 10.1001/jama.300.12.1423

[10] Rajan S, Folke F, Hansen SM, Hansen CM, Kragholm K, Gerds TA, et al. Incidence and survival outcome according to heart rhythm during resuscitation attempt in out-of-hospital cardiac arrest patients with presumed cardiac etiology. Resuscitation. 2017;**114**(5):157-163. DOI: 10.1016/j.resuscitation.2016.12.021

[11] Stokes NA, Scapigliati A, Trammell AR, Parish DC. The effect of the AED and AED programs on survival of individuals, groups and populations. Prehospital and Disaster Medicine. 2012;**27**(5):419-424. DOI: 10.1017/S1049023X12001197

[12] Meaney PA, Nadkarni VM, Kern KB, Indik JH, Halperin HR, Berg RA. Rhythms and outcomes of adult in-hospital cardiac arrest. Critical Care Medicine. 2010;**38**(1):101-108. DOI: 10.1097/CCM.0b013e3181b43282

[13] Sandroni C, Nolan J, Cavallaro F, Antonelli M. In-hospital cardiac arrest: Incidence, prognosis and possible measures to improve survival. Intensive Care Medicine. 2007;**33**(2):237-245. DOI: 10.1007/s00134-006-0326-z

[14] Girotra S, Nallamothu BK, Spertus JA, Li Y, Krumholz HM, Chan PS, et al. Trends in survival after in-hospital cardiac arrest. The New England Journal of Medicine. 2012;**367**(20):1912-1920. DOI: 10.1056/NEJMoa1109148

[15] Bergum D, Haugen BO, Nordseth T, Mjølstad OC, Skogvoll E. Recognizing the causes of in-hospital cardiac arrest—A survival benefit. Resuscitation. 2015;**97**:91-96. DOI: 10.1016/j.resuscitation.2015.09.395

[16] Bergum D, Nordseth T, Mjølstad OC, Skogvoll E, Haugen BO. Causes of in-hospital cardiac arrest—Incidences and rate of recognition. Resuscitation. 2015;**87**:63-68. DOI: 10.1016/j.resuscitation.2014.11.007

[17] Nolan JP, Soar J, Smith GB, Gwinnutt C, Parrott F, Power S, et al. Incidence and outcome of in-hospital cardiac arrest in the United Kingdom. Resuscitation. 2014;**85**(8):987-992. DOI: 10.1016/j.resuscitation.2014.04.002

[18] Radeschi G, Mina A, Berta G, Fassiola A, Roasio A, Urso F, et al. Incidence and outcome of in-hospital cardiac arrest in Italy: A multicentre observational study in the Piedmont Region. Resuscitation. 2017;**119**:48-55. DOI: 10.1016/j.resuscitation.2017.06.020

[19] Caffrey SL, Willoughby PJ, Pepe PE, Becker LB. Public use automated external defibrillators. The New England Journal of Medicine. 2002;**347**(16):1242-1247. DOI: 10.1056/NEJMoa020932

[20] Hazinski MF, Nadkarni VM, Hickey RW, O'Connor R, Becker LB, Zaritsky A. Major changes in the 2005 AHA Guidelines for CPR and ECC: Reaching the tipping point for change. Circulation. 2005;**112** (24 Suppl):IV206-IV211. DOI: 10.1161/CIRCULATIONAHA.105.170809

[21] Kuzovlev AN, Abdusalamov SN, Kuzmichev KA. Assessment of the quality of basic and advanced resuscitation in a multifield hospital (simulation course). Obshchaya Reanimatologiya (General Reanimatology). 2016;**12**(6):27-38. DOI: 10.15360/1813-9779-2016-6-27-38. [In Russ., In Engl.]

[22] Wissenberg M, Lippert FK, Folke F, Weeke P, Hansen CM, Christensen EF, et al. Association of national initiatives to improve cardiac arrest management with rates of bystander intervention and patient survival after out-of-hospital cardiac arrest. JAMA. 2013;**310**(13):1377-1384. DOI: 10.1001/jama.2013.278483

[23] Hasselqvist-Ax I, Riva G, Herlitz J, Rosenqvist M, Hollenberg J, Nordberg P, et al. Early cardiopulmonary resuscitation in out-of-hospital cardiac arrest. The New England Journal of Medicine. 2015;**372**(24):2307-2315. DOI: 10.1056/NEJMoa1405796

[24] Hostler D, Everson-Stewart S, Rea TD, et al. Effect of real-time feedback during cardiopulmonary resuscitation outside hospital: Prospective, cluster randomised trial. British Medical Journal. 2011;**342**:d512. DOI: 10.1136/bmj.d512

[25] Stiell IG, Brown SP, Christenson J, et al. What is the role of chest compression depth during out-of-hospital cardiac arrest resuscitation? Critical Care Medicine. 2012;**40**:1192-1198. DOI: 10.1097/CCM.0b013e31823bc8bb

[26] Stiell IG, Brown SP, Nichol G, et al. What is the optimal chest compression depth during out-of-hospital cardiac arrest resuscitation of adult patients? Circulation. 2014;**130**:1962-1970. DOI: 10.1161/CIRCULATIONAHA.114.008671

[27] Hellevuo H, Sainio M, Nevalainen R, et al. Deeper chest compression—More complications for cardiac

arrest patients? Resuscitation. 2013;**84**:760-765. DOI: 10.1016/j.resuscitation.2013.02.015

[28] Idris AH, Guffey D, Pepe PE, et al. Chest compression rates and survival following out-of-hospital cardiac arrest. Critical Care Medicine. 2015;**43**:840-848. DOI: 10.1097/CCM.0000000000000824

[29] Idris AH, Guffey D, Aufderheide TP, et al. Relationship between chest compression rates and outcomes from cardiac arrest. Circulation. 2012;**125**:3004-3012. DOI: 10.1161/CIRCULATIONAHA.111.059535

[30] Aufderheide T, Pirrallo R, Yannopoulos D, Klein JP, vonBriesen C, Sparks CW, et al. Incomplete chest wall decompression: A clinical evaluation of CPR performance by trained laypersons and an assessment of alternative manual chest compression-decompression techniques. Resuscitation. 2006;**71**(3):341-351

[31] Kovacs A, Vadeboncoeur T, Stolz U, Spaite D, Irisawa T, Silver A, et al. Chest compression release velocity: Association with survival and favorable neurologic outcome after out-of-hospital cardiac arrest. Resuscitation. 2015;**92**:107-114. DOI: 10.1016/j.resuscitation.2015.04.026

[32] Weisfeldt ML, Sitlani CM, Ornato JP, Rea T, Aufderheide TP, Davis D, et al. Survival after application of automatic external defibrillators before arrival of the emergency medical system: Evaluation in the resuscitation outcomes consortium population of 21 million. Journal of the American College of Cardiology. 2010;**55**(16):1713-1720. DOI: 10.1016/j.jacc.2009.11.077.

[33] Agerskov M, Nielsen AM, Hansen CM, Hansen MB, Lippert FK, Wissenberg M, et al. Public access defibrillation: Great benefit and potential but infrequently used. Resuscitation. 2015;**96**:53-58. DOI: 10.1016/j.resuscitation.2015.07.021

[34] Lijovic M, Bernard S, Nehme Z, Walker T, Smith K, Victorian Ambulance Cardiac Arrest Registry Steering Committee. Public access defibrillation—Results from the Victorian Ambulance Cardiac Arrest Registry. Resuscitation. 2014;**85**(12):1739-1744. DOI: 10.1016/j.resuscitation.2014.10.005

[35] Kitamura T, Kiyohara K, Sakai T, Matsuyama T, Hatakeyama T, Shimamoto T, et al. Public-access defibrillation and out-of-hospital cardiac arrest in Japan. The New England Journal of Medicine. 2016;**375**(17):1649-1659. DOI: 10.1056/NEJMsa1600011

[36] Ringh M, Rosenqvist M, Hollenberg J, Jonsson M, Fredman D, Nordberg P, et al. Mobilephone dispatch of laypersons for CPR in out-of-hospital cardiac arrest. The New England Journal of Medicine. 2015;**372**:2316-2325. DOI: 10.1056/NEJMoa1406038

[37] Kudenchuk PJ, Redshaw JD, Stubbs BA, Fahrenbruch CE, Dumas F, Phelps R, et al. Impact of changes in resuscitation practice on survival and neurological outcome after out-of-hospital cardiac arrest resulting from nonshockable arrhythmias. Circulation. 2012;**125**(14):1787-1794. DOI: 10.1161/CIRCULATIONAHA.111.064873

[38] Steinberg MT, Olsen JA, Brunborg C, Persse D, Sterz F, Lozano M Jr, et al. Minimizing pre-shock chest compression pauses in a cardiopulmonary resuscitation cycle by performing an earlier rhythm analysis. Resuscitation. 2015;**87**:33-37. DOI: 10.1016/j.resuscitation.2014.11.012

[39] Song KJ, Shin SD, Park CB, Kim JY, Kim DK, Kim CH, et al. Dispatcher-assisted bystander cardiopulmonary

resuscitation in a metropolitan city: A before-after population-based study. Resuscitation. 2014;**85**(1):34-41. DOI: 10.1016/j.resuscitation.2013.06.004

[40] Forcina MS, Farhat AY, O'Neil WW, Haines DE. Cardiac arrest survival after implementation of automated external defibrillator technology in the in-hospital setting. Critical Care Medicine. 2009;**37**(4):1229-1236. DOI: 10.1097/CCM.0b013e3181960ff3

[41] Smith RJ, Hickey BB, Santamaria JD. Automated external defibrillators and survival after in-hospital cardiac arrest: Early experience at an Australian teaching hospital. Critical Care and Resuscitation. 2009;**11**(4):261-265

[42] Smith RJ, Hickey BB, Santamaria JD. Automated external defibrillators and in-hospital cardiac arrest: Patient survival and device performance at an Australian teaching hospital. Resuscitation. 2011;**82**(12):1537-1542. DOI: 10.1016/j.resuscitation.2011.06.025

[43] Chan PS, Krumholz HM, Spertus JA, Jones PG, Cram P, Berg RA, et al. Automated external defibrillators and survival after in-hospital cardiac arrest. JAMA. 2010;**304**(19):2129-2136. DOI: 10.1001/jama.2010.1576

[44] Gibbison B, Soar J. Automated external defibrillator use for in-hospital cardiac arrest is not associated with improved survival. Evidence-Based Medicine. 2011;**16**(3):95-96. DOI: 10.1136/ebm1195

[45] Husain S, Eisenberg M. Police AED programs: A systematic review and meta-analysis. Resuscitation. 2013;**84**(9):1184-1191. DOI: 10.1016/j.resuscitation.2013.03.040

[46] Schober A, Sterz F, Laggner AN, Poppe M, Sulzgruber P, Lobmeyr E, et al. Admission of out-of-hospital cardiac arrest victims to a high volume cardiac arrest center is linked to improved outcome. Resuscitation. 2016;**106**:42-48. DOI: 10.1016/j.resuscitation.2016.06.021

[47] Elmer J, Rittenberger JC, Coppler PJ, Guyette FX, Doshi AA, Callaway CW, et al. Long-term survival benefit from treatment at a specialty center after cardiac arrest. Resuscitation. 2016;**108**:48-53. DOI: 10.1016/j.resuscitation.2016.09.008

[48] Bækgaard JS, Viereck S, Møller TP, Ersbøll AK, Lippert F, Folke F. The effects of public access defibrillation on survival after out-of-hospital cardiac arrest: A systematic review of observational studies. Circulation. 2017;**136**(10):954-965. DOI: 10.1161/CIRCULATIONAHA.117.029067

[49] Baekgaard JS, Viereck S, Møller TP, Ersbøll AK, Lippert F, Folke F. Response by Baekgaard et al. to letters regarding article, "The effects of public access defibrillation on survival after out-of-hospital cardiac arrest: A systematic review of observational studies". Circulation. 2018;**137**(15):1650-1651. DOI: 10.1161/CIRCULATIONAHA.117.032513

[50] Srinivasan NT, Schilling RJ. Sudden cardiac death and arrhythmias. Arrhythmia & Electrophysiology Review. 2018;7(2):111-117. DOI: 10.15420/aer.2018:15:2